Skincare Ethnic Beauty, Acne, Ageing, Cellulite, Pigmentation, Tattoo Regret, and Unwanted Hair

Ancient Rituals, Modern Myths, and Future Realities

Katie Lewis and Jarrett Zapletal

Disclaimer

The authors of this book are not, nor claiming to be, doctors/physicians, nurses, physician's assistants, advanced practice nurses, or any other type of medical professional ('medical provider'), psychiatrist, psychologist, therapist, counsellor, or social worker ('mental health provider'), registered dietician or licensed nutritionist, or member of the clergy.

We are not providing healthcare, medical or nutritional therapy services, or attempting to diagnose, treat, prevent, or cure any physical, mental, or emotional issue, disease, or condition. The information provided in or through this website pertaining to your health or wellness, exercise, relationships, business/career choices, finances, or any other aspect of your life is not intended to be a substitute for the professional medical advice, diagnosis, and/or treatment provided by your own medical provider or mental health provider. You agree and acknowledge that we are not providing medical, mental health, or religious advice in any way.

Always seek the advice of your own medical provider or mental health provider regarding any questions or concerns about your specific health or any medications, herbs, or supplements you are currently taking before implementing any recommendations or suggestions from our website. Do not disregard medical advice or delay seeking medical advice because of information you have read in this book/audiobook, ebook, or website. Do not start or stop taking any medications without speaking to your own medical provider or mental health provider. If you have or suspect a medical or mental health problem, contact your own medical provider or mental health provider promptly. The information contained in this book/audiobook, ebook, and website has not been evaluated by Health U.K. or the Food and Drug Administration.

Contents

Introduction

Take care of your mind, body, and soul, nourish them and keep them young and happy, and with the wisdom that grows with age, you will love getting old.

With these words, Jarrett Zapletal, co-author of this skin guide, summarises his view on ageing and life. Jarrett represents a new generation of men who regard fitness and skincare as part of staying healthy and having optimal quality of life. He personally experienced how a healthy lifestyle, especially a diet of predominantly fresh vegetables and herbs, changed his life. He now actively promotes living healthily as the first line of defence in improving skin health, preventing premature ageing, and enduring quality of life.

Katie Lewis is a trained cosmetologist who, during her years of practice, realised how deeply clients with skin problems suffered emotionally. In her long career, she often treated desperate and deeply unhappy people: teenagers with cystic acne and new moms with unsightly brown pigmentation marks. All too often, post-menopausal women came to her for help when they could no longer hide ageing skin. But it was the needs of transgender women that grabbed her heart. Katie specialises in electrolysis and now helps transgender people suffering from unwanted hair to transition to smoother skin and greater self-acceptance.

Katie and Jarrett are deeply aware that people with skin problems and premature ageing often hide their devastation behind a mask – sometimes pretending not to care, other times using heavy make-up, and even isolating themselves from social interaction.

The authors pride themselves on staying up to date with the latest scientific developments on treatments for skin problems. They highlight how skincare has benefitted from science and medical research since mediaeval times. You will also get a glimpse of the future of skincare, when health is a prerequisite for good skin and technology will increasingly help you make the best of what you have.

They do not promote any brand and are not sponsored by any cosmeceutical retailer.

In this guide, Katie and Jarrett help you to identify your skin type, which is vital for treating it correctly. You will learn which ingredients are effective and when to seek professional help. They want you to understand how your skin works: its anatomy (the different layers and their components) and physiology (each component's function). You will also learn to recognise empty marketing buzzwords and false claims. This book will guide you to distinguish between myths and science-based facts.

They will help you identify which lifestyle choices contribute to your skin problems and might be ageing you prematurely. You will see how an unhealthy diet, lack of exercise, smoking, and excessive drinking directly damage your skin's natural regeneration.

The skin is our biggest organ; it is alive, an incredibly hard worker, and very intelligent. It reveals gender, race, age, and health and shows the individual's level of personal care. It surrounds and protects the body from many daily dangers: injuries, heat, cold, pollution, and the sun.

Although often not realised, the skin is a powerful storyteller. When embarrassed, the skin is flushed; when in shock, the skin turns ashen. When unwell, the skin tone is dull. The skin will even reveal when one is emotionally down. It is a sure giveaway of prolonged stress, smoking, living unhealthily, and emotional, physical, or alcohol abuse.

When someone touches you, your skin reacts instinctively: sometimes with pleasure, sometimes in disgust. It often reveals more than you would want the world to know.

Wonderful though the skin might be, it might cause much pain, ruin your self-esteem, rob you of confidence, and even take away the joy of living. People with skin problems often experience acute embarrassment and emotional trauma.

Every life stage has its own skin challenges: acne, hyperpigmentation, unwanted hair, and premature ageing. Every skin colour has problems. Light skin is more prone to sun damage, wrinkling, and age spots. Olive and darker skin might not age quickly, but hyperpigmentation causes heartbreak – brown patches and dark rings around the eyes, skin tags, and enlarged pores.

But there is hope. Even if your skin is damaged and neglected, you can still do a lot to improve skin quality and your appearance. An overview of skincare through the ages proves that the desire to look one's best is as old as time itself, and that inner beauty goes hand in hand with personal care and well-being. This skincare guide will help you to do just that: You might have left youth and its fresh beauty behind long ago, but you can still take care of your skin and your life.

This guide will help you determine your unique beauty irrespective of race, age, or wealth. Be warned, though: Despite marketing promises, results are seldom instant. Skincare is much more than expensive creams and advanced treatments; it starts with how you live.

This guide is the ideal companion as you journey through the many beauty challenges every stage of life brings.

Part 1: Knowledge Is Power – Also in Skincare

Chapter 1:
The Anatomy and Physiology of the Skin

Beauty is a fragile gift.

'Beauty is a fragile gift,' said Publius Ovidius Naso, better known as Ovid, many centuries ago. His wise words on the fragility of beauty ring true even today and are particularly true of the human skin.

The skin is a complex organ, the biggest in the human body, making up about 15% of the body's weight (Kolarsick et al., 2011). You have around 19 million tiny cells in every square inch of your skin, 1,000 nerve endings, and 20 blood vessels (Cleveland Clinic, n.d.).

So what do human organs do, and why are our organs so important?

Biologists define an organ as a collection of tissues that form a structure or a unit with a specific function in the body. The definition explains the name of this chapter. The anatomy of the skin describes the *structure* of the different parts of the skin. Physiology describes the *function* of the skin and how it works.

The skin fits the definition of an organ perfectly. It consists of three layers: the epidermis, dermis, and subcutaneous fat layer. Each of these layers is uniquely constructed with specific functions. If we leave aside the fact that your skin is the package you present to the world, the skin performs several vital biological functions:

- It protects the body from potentially harmful microbes and tiny living cells. Microbes can be harmless but can also cause infections or diseases.

- It helps to regulate body temperature through hair coverings and sweat glands. These ensure that the human body can tolerate temperature fluctuations without being harmed.

- It is responsible for the touch sense. Without your skin, you would never feel the softness of a baby's hands or the mildness of a spring day on your cheeks.

The skin is sensitive yet strong. It amazingly regenerates itself regularly and, consequently, can benefit from the right type of treatment. The success of cosmetic products will greatly depend on how effectively they can enhance the function of the skin's different layers and components.

Your skin is truly a miracle, as it is alive and continuously forming new cells. These cells start life in the basal layer of the epidermis and are pushed to the surface, where they die. The miracle of the human skin does not stop there. The dead cells, or corneocytes, are shed and replaced by new ones in a process called desquamation. Desquamation refreshes the skin continuously as new cells come to the surface.

Knowing your skin will help you to make the best of it and improve your appearance and confidence. The better you know your skin and its complexities, the better equipped you will be to care for it correctly. Don't expect results immediately. Your body is not a computer in fast-forward mode, but you will look and feel better over time.

If you already regard your skin as a beauty asset, more knowledge will help you to stay abreast of the newest ingredients and technology in skincare. However, if your skin is the cause of embarrassment or pain, this book will help you identify the cause of your skin problem. Moreover, you will get advice on addressing your skin issue with the latest and most advanced treatments.

The Epidermis

The epidermis may be as thin as the softest paper, but it is remarkably strong. It is thinnest on your eyelid and much thicker on your palms and the soles of your feet.

The epidermis consists of several sub-layers. Do not get confused: The skin has three layers, and the epidermis has four sub-layers. As you use this guide, you will find that the very outermost layer of the epidermis, the stratum corneum (SC), is the focus of skincare.

You might wonder why the dead cells of the stratum corneum are so important in skincare. Despite what advertisers want you to believe, external skincare products do not go any deeper than the outer layer of the epidermis. The reason is that the cells in the uppermost layer of the skin are as hard as bricks and difficult to penetrate. By no means should you give up on skincare, though. The right skincare products interact with the moisture in the stratum corneum and help to seal it in.

Let us look at the three sub-layers of the epidermis. The stratum corneum, the outermost layer of the epidermis, forms the skin barrier. The skin barrier is another term you will repeatedly hear in this book. Just to confirm, the cells in the stratum corneum are dead. Yes, they are dead, but you still have to moisturise them.

The other three layers of the epidermis – the granular, basal, and squamous – are alive. Even though they cannot benefit from topical lotions, they play a vital role in skin quality.

The cells in the epidermis are predominantly keratinocytes with fewer dendritic cells.

- Keratinocytes contain keratin, a key ingredient in cosmetics and hair products. Keratin is a type of protein, and cytes is the scientific word for cells. Keratin is fibrous and the main component in the epidermis, hair, and nails. Keratinocytes form a protective layer on your skin, and together they make up the backbone of your epidermis.

- Dendritic cells are vital in the skin's immune responses. They are also found in the lining of the nose, lungs, stomach, and intestines.

HUMAN SKIN

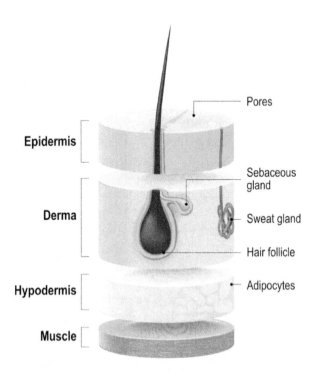

Pores

Epidermis

Sebaceous gland

Derma

Sweat gland

Hair follicle

Hypodermis

Adipocytes

Muscle

Regeneration of the Epidermis

Remember, the epidermis has its own sub-layers. These layers are dynamic and undergo constant regeneration. In younger people, it takes the cells around 28 days to move from the basal layer to the topmost dead layer (stratum corneum) (Kolarsick et al., 2011). This process slows down with age, though.

Skin regeneration in women 50 and older might take up to 84 days, depending on diet, skincare routine, hydration levels, and environmental factors (Walters, 2022).

Keep this timespan in mind when you squeeze a pimple. Squeezing damages the fragile cells in your epidermis, and the chances are good that the surrounding area might get infected. Even if you get the pus out, it leaves a red, inflamed, and unsightly wound. Healing depends on new cell formation. It means you have to wait anyhow for the damaged cells to be shed and the new ones to migrate to the surface. Instead of forcing the zit to pop, you delay the healing.

As the new cells move from the basal layer, they form attachment plates that interact and connect with other plates. These connections strengthen the skin and help form the structure and shape of your face.

As the cells migrate upward, they lose moisture and eventually die. At this stage, they become hard and are called corneocytes. Corneocytes might be dead, but they can absorb small amounts of moisture that keep your skin hydrated.

Scientists and cosmetic researchers are constantly researching and developing products based on the epidermis's ability to renew itself by moving old cells to the surface. Through the centuries, and especially during the last decades, cosmetic research has benefitted immensely from medical research, specifically regarding wound healing.

The Basal Layer at the Bottom of the Epidermis

New cell formation occurs in the basal layer at the bottom of the epidermis. Cell regeneration in the basal layer starts when the keratinocytes (the cells containing the protein keratin) divide rapidly. New cells are pushed upward to make space for even newer cells.

Distributed between the keratinocytes are melanocytes, cells with very different functions. In a complicated process (given here in a simplified version), melanocytes produce melanin, a pigment that contains amino acids.

The colour of your skin depends largely on the amount of melanin produced by the melanocytes. The amount of melanin in your skin also determines whether you tan brown or just turn red. It even determines whether you will develop freckles. Remember, your skin colour is also influenced by the amount of time you spend in the sun, your hormones, and your genes.

The melanocytes produce melanin in the basal layer. The melanin then moves into the keratinocytes. Melanin's primary function is to protect you from the harmful effect of ultraviolet radiation.

The Squamous Layer of the Epidermis

The squamous layer is right above the basal layer and is the thickest part of the epidermis. As the name indicates, the cells in this layer look like fish scales. The cells in the squamous layer also attach to other cells to form a protective barrier against injuries and physical stress.

The Granular Layer of the Epidermis

The granular layer is the top *living layer* of the epidermis. The granular layer on the palms and feet is understandably thicker than on the face.

The cells in the granular layer consist mostly of soft keratin in contrast to the hard keratin in hair and nails. As the cell moves through the granular layer, it loses moisture, becomes harder, and ends up dry and dead in the stratum corneum.

The Stratum Corneum

We are now back at the *topmost layer, the stratum corneum, with dead cells*. As stated earlier, most cosmetic products don't go deeper than the stratum corneum. If these cells are dead, does it make any sense to feed them with expensive moisturisers? Would petroleum jelly not protect the skin as effectively from dehydration?

The answer is undeniable: Yes. You have to moisturise your skin diligently. Modern moisturisers and serums are scientifically formulated to prevent dehydration. Also, many modern products contain humectants, an agent that retains moisture in the dead cells of the stratum corneum. And yes, petroleum jelly is useful to keep the skin's natural moisture intact.

The cornified cells in the stratum corneum are vital to protect the skin, as they retain moisture and prevent harmful substances from penetrating the skin. Furthermore, these cells are programmed to die, a process called programmed death. Programmed death illustrates how intricate and special the human skin is.

Usually, dead tissue affects the neighbouring tissue as well, but in programmed death, the cell dies without any damage to the surrounding cells. On top of that, as the cell dies, a new one takes its place. Skincare products target the newer cells, as they can absorb moisture and plumb out and make your skin look fresher.

Theoretically, harmful microbes can enter the skin through the tiny openings between the dead corneocytes and also through the openings of the hair follicles. But the body has a perfect defence system. Lipids (the oils in the skin) gather in these mini-openings between the corneocytes, and sebum fills the hair follicles. Together they form a natural barrier to keep harmful molecules and dirt out.

Unfortunately, this barrier also prevents cosmetic ingredients from entering the granular, squamous, or basal layers of the epidermis. In an ideal world, one would have wished for the skincare products to penetrate the skin deeply, even reaching the dermis where collagen is formed. Unfortunately, skincare creams do not even get to the basal layer to form new cells.

Several cosmetic houses recently claimed that newly developed products contain peptides and that their products stimulate collagen production. It is exciting news, but unfortunately, scientific findings must be supported by large-scale studies and peer-evaluated publications in scientific journals. Up till now, not enough scientific evidence is available. Nonetheless, the possibility that peptides could stimulate the production of collagen and elastin is generally welcomed. It is discussed in more detail in the chapter on skin products and key ingredients.

It is essential to distinguish between cosmetic products and medical treatments such as nicotine and hormonal patches. These patches do eventually reach the bloodstream and have long-term consequences. Cosmetic products, though, have only a short-term localised effect on the skin.

Cosmeceutical research is a relatively new field that combines physics, chemistry, and biology in the quest for cosmetics that also have a therapeutic effect on the skin. As research continues, we can expect exciting new products and technology.

Epidermal Appendages

Hair, nails, and the various sweat glands form part of the human skin's epidermal appendages. They are interesting features, as they grow from the outside inward. The process starts already during the embryo stage in the womb.

A woman's hair is called her crowning glory, and well-kept nails ooze sophistication, but hair and nails are much more than just aesthetic features. They perform vital functions in the body.

Sweat Glands

Sweat glands might be less glamorous, but they are still vital in our bodies. Humans have three diverse types of sweat glands, and those on the face are called eccrine sweat glands. We usually associate sweat with an unpleasant odour, but the eccrine (facial) sweat glands' secretion is odourless.

(Do not confuse the eccrine glands with the apocrine glands in the armpits. The latter glands are the smelly culprits, as they secrete a thick fluid that, when it comes into contact with the skin's surface, causes an unpleasant odour.)

The clear sweat produced by the facial eccrine glands is good for the skin in more than one way. It helps to cool the body, especially during exercise and on hot days. Evaporation causes cooling, and the body cools down when the sweat evaporates.

Sweat has some interesting additional benefits for your skin. It has high water content and thus hydrates the skin. It also contains urea and uric acid, good moisturisers for dry skin.

Furthermore, the minerals and salt in the sweat serve as an exfoliate, and they naturally clean the skin. They wash bacteria, dirt particles, and impurities from the pores. It rids the skin of toxins, and the immune system is automatically boosted.

If you are still not convinced that sweat can be good for your skin, check your skin after a strenuous exercise session. You will be glowing; your skin will look hydrated and fresher.

Hair Follicles

Did you always want thicker hair and tried many products that promised you just that? Here is the bad news. You are born with a specific number of hair follicles that appear in a distinctive pattern over your head and body. It is a given, and nothing you can do can change your hair type or the potential number of hair on your head. (However, if you want to get rid of excess hair, Chapter 7 tells you everything about electrolysis and why you should not be scared of it.)

The tiny hair follicle is a miracle in itself. It might be small, but it is intricately constructed with several components. The sebaceous gland develops as a tiny bud at the bottom of the follicle, but more on the sebaceous gland later.

Small Muscle Bundle

Below the sebaceous gland is a small and smooth muscle bundle attached to the follicle's root sheath. The tiny muscle bundles contain stem cells that have the ability to regenerate the hair follicle. Thus, if you pluck out the hair with the follicle, the muscle bundle stays behind and, consequently, a new follicle will regrow. It might take a while, but in the end, your hair follicle will be regenerated and new hair will grow because of another tiny miracle at the bottom of the hair follicle, the hair bulb.

Hair Bulb

The hair bulb holds even more surprises. While the muscle bundle is responsible for the regrowth of the hair follicle, the bulb is responsible for the growth of the hair shaft. The hair bulb's matrix cells proliferate rapidly, producing the hair shaft, its inner root sheath, and its outer root sheath.

That long, glossy hair you are so proud of (or desire so intensely) stems from the tiny bulbs at the bottom of the hair follicles. The shape and size of the inner root sheath determine the structure of your hair texture – straight, wavy, or curly.

Hair grows in three phases. During the first anagen phase, the hair grows actively. The growth phase can last between three to five years. After the growth stage follows the catagen phase, when the follicle shrinks. The hair separates from the follicle but stays in place. During the last phase, or telogen phase, the hair follicle takes a rest for a couple of months (WebMD, 2010).

Getting grey hair is part of getting older, and the origin of your grey hair lies in the hair bulb. It's time for a bit of simplified science again: The hair bulb contains melanocytes, the same cells as in the basal layer. As the name indicates, melanocytes contain melanin, contributing to skin and hair colour. However, with age, the melanocytes produce less and less melanin, and the hair becomes gradually lighter. Consequently, as the melanocytes age, you end up with grey hair.

Fortunately, modern hair dyes can solve the problem. Alternatively, you can enjoy the softness that your particular shade of grey brings to your features. Once the greying has started, the process cannot be turned around, and you will never regain your original hair colour.

Redheads are unique, as they have a genetic variant that produces more red melanin to make a redhead stand out among the rest of the population. Redheads, celebrate your uniqueness!

Nails

Your nails were not meant to be decorations but are there to protect the fingers and toes. Nonetheless, polished and neat nails do round off a well-kept appearance. The opposite is also true; your nails are a sure giveaway if you don't take care of yourself.

Nails consist primarily of keratin, and, as we know, keratin strengthens your skin, hair, and nails. The visible part of your nail is dead, similar to the hair shaft and the stratum corneum, the outermost layer of your skin. Therefore, you can cut your nails without any pain. However, you have some feeling in the nails because of the nerve endings in the dermis directly under the nail.

Also, under the nail bed, you have tiny capillaries that feed the nail bed. Nails grow faster in summer than in the winter. Interestingly, the nails on your dominant hand grow faster than the nails on the other hand. Scientists believe that increased blood flow to the dominant hand stimulates nail growth.

Look out:

- Be aware of colour changes in the nails, as a change in colour might indicate an underlying health problem such as fungi, thyroid dysfunction, diabetes, or psoriasis.

- Your grandmother was wrong when she said calcium shortage caused her white spots. The white is caused by injuries, mostly so small that you don't even notice it.

- Many women are worried about the horizontal lines on their nails. They are the result of stress and, though harmless, are a warning that you should take care of yourself for a change. Also, although nail-biting is harmless, it is unhygienic and should be avoided.

- Well-kept nails don't have to be painted. Unpolished nails can still be well-kept, clean, and attractive. Moreover, your nails must get enough breathing time. Nail polish and polish removers damage the nails when used consistently. Thus, give your nails a chance to recover.

- Handle your cuticles with care. They protect the nail base; therefore, don't cut away too harshly.

Sebaceous Glands

The sebaceous glands are the last but not the least of the appendages of the epidermis to discuss. As you can see from the names, these glands produce sebum, a natural lipid moisturising skin. The sebocytes produce sebum and, like keratinocytes, sebocytes are also programmed to die. As the sebocytes dissolve, they release sebum into the hair follicle.

The sebum is pushed to the surface as natural lubrication for the skin and the scalp. But if too much sebum is released, you might develop a skin problem.

The sebaceous glands are vital in all types of acne and can cause havoc on the skin. Chapter 6 discusses these glands and their role in acne in detail.

Dermo-Epidermal Junction

The epidermis and the dermis meet at the dermo-epidermal junction. It is a multi-layered membrane that holds the epidermis and the dermis together. It supports the epidermis and plays a major role in getting oxygen, nutrients, and fluids to the epidermis. The membrane is porous, which allows movement for nourishment upward and waste matter downward.

Additionally, the dermo-epidermal membrane strengthens the skin and offers protection against injuries from the outside.

The Dermis

The dermis is the largest component of the skin and further supports the epidermis. It forms a cushion for the epidermis to rest on, thus protecting the fragile epidermis.

Although cosmetic products do not penetrate the dermis, a healthy dermis is vital for skin health. It feeds the epidermis and protects it. It contributes to the skin's pliability and elasticity, binds water, regulates temperature, and allows for your touch sense.

The dermis consists of a network of connective tissue and blood vessels. The epidermis does not have any blood vessels, so it depends on the dermis for nourishment and waste removal.

The dermis and the epidermis (except for the outermost stratum corneum) are living parts of your skin. They interact with each other through the dermo-epidermal junction. The epidermal appendages (hair, nails, sweat, and sebaceous glands discussed above) are part of the cooperation and interaction between these two layers of the skin.

The dermis is particularly interesting as it consists mainly of collagen, elastin, and hyaluronic acid, buzzwords in modern skincare.

Natural Substances in the Dermis

Collagen

Collagen is the principal protein in the dermis and forms about 70% of the dermis (Kolarsick, 2011). Collagen is not exclusively found in the dermis. The tendons, ligaments, and bone linings also have this type of protein. It confirms how important collagen is, in and for the human body.

Collagen gives strength and adds resilience to the skin, as it consists of protein fibres that form a connective network called fibroblasts. The network (together with other skin components) is responsible for the architectural framework of the body (Alberts, 2002). Think of the fibroblasts giving shape to your skin as your teeth give form to your mouth.

Fibroblasts play a significant role in wound healing. When the skin is injured, the fibroblasts around the area proliferate and produce large numbers of special cells that promote healing and break down the fibrin clot.

Like many other cells in human skin, collagen cells are not static but are constantly changing. In layperson's terms, they get old and disintegrate, but new cells form continuously. The skin is indeed a living and dynamic organ, a good reason for you to look after it. Collagen in skin products and collagen supplements are discussed in the following two chapters.

Elastin

Elastin is made up of different protein molecules and, true to its name, elastin can stretch and shrink. It is why your skin returns to its shape when it is stretched or pinched.

Unfortunately, with age, the skin's elasticity reduces as less elastin is produced. Too much sun exposure causes ultraviolet radiation that destroys elastin production, a process known as photoaging. If you care for your skin, it is vital to prevent sun damage at all costs. You cannot stop the natural ageing process, but you can do a lot to prevent sun damage. You can read more about photoaging and hyperpigmentation in Chapter 5 and Chapter 9.

Hyaluronic Acid

Hyaluronic acid is not a protein but a natural water-binding substance in the dermis, also found in the eyes. Although not as plentiful as collagen or elastin, hyaluronic acid is vital for retaining moisture in the skin.

It controls tissue hydration by retaining large quantities of water. Hyaluronic acid is a natural lubricator in soft tissue.

Medical professionals use hyaluronic acid in wound healing, and cosmetic science has benefitted significantly from medical research in this field. It has anti-inflammatory and antibacterial properties. When the skin is injured, the surrounding cells increase the production of hyaluronic acid to help in the healing process.

More Structures in the Dermis

Blood vessels

The dermis has a network of blood vessels. The blood vessels in the uppermost layer of the dermis are tiny capillaries. The blood vessels deeper in the dermis and the dermis-subcutaneous junction are more extensive and are supplied with fresh blood by larger blood vessels.

It is crucial to remember that the epidermis does not have any blood vessels. The epidermis depends on the small capillaries in the upper part of the dermis for a supply of oxygen, nourishment, and fluids. These small capillaries also remove the waste from the epidermis. Following the rule of nature, oxygen and nutrients move from the higher concentration in the capillaries to the 'empty' cells in the epidermis. In the same way, the waste is channelled via the capillaries to the blood vessels and the kidneys.

The network of superficial and deeper blood vessels in the dermis is vital in regulating the body's temperature. The skin does not regulate the temperature in isolation, though. It works with the hypothalamus situated in the brain, another example of how wonderfully intricate the human body is.

The hypothalamus tries to keep your body temperature at around 37°C. When the body gets too hot, the hypothalamus instructs the capillaries in the dermis to widen. More blood moves into the capillaries and heat is released into the air; consequently, the body cools down. When the body gets too cold, the hypothalamus sends the opposite message. The capillaries constrict, the blood flow increases, and heat is contained.

If you have ever wondered where hot flushes originate, recent research links menopausal hot flushes to changes in the capillaries (Hazell, 2011).

Muscles in the Dermis

The facial muscles are controlled by a cranial nerve that splits into several smaller nerves, which then go to different facial areas. These nerves allow humans to express a range of feelings and emotions. And when you don't want to show your true feelings, you can cleverly control these nerves to hide your true thoughts.

You might wonder why information on facial expression is included in a skincare guide. Have you ever seen a beautiful grumpy woman? How you feel and how you view the world shows on your face. When you smile from your soul, you are much more attractive than a forced or false smile. Your facial expressions reveal your emotions and mental state. However, in unguarded moments, your face might give away what you want to hide.

Facial expressions are pretty much an international language. A smile is a smile, whether you are friendly in Samoa or Saudi. A frown is a frown, regardless of your foul mood in France or Finland. Smiling and frowning are only two of the endless messages we send others without speaking a word. Furthermore, you might smile with just one corner of the mouth, or wide and with an open mouth and eyes. It is the reason why statistics on how many muscles you use for smiling differ so much.

Your facial muscles originate from the skull and protrude into the dermis. They work together to bring movement to your cheeks, eyebrows, eyelids, forehead, upper and lower lips, nose, and nostrils. And if you are exceptional, even your ears! Only between 10 and 20% of the population can wiggle their ears (Joi, 2009).

Your facial muscles are not only involved in expression but also assist in determining personal appearance. They protect the eyes and play a role in talking, singing, and eating – they even prevent drooling.

Mast Cells

Mast cells are the dermis's resident anti-inflammatory fighters. They help in the fight against acne, and you will learn more about mast cells in the chapter on acne. They release histamine to counteract allergic reactions and kick in immediately after an injury. Mast cells also stimulate the growth of keratinocytes.

The Hypodermis, or Subcutaneous Fat Layer

Right at the bottom of the skin is a fatty layer called the hypodermis. There are few things women like less than fat. Fat is regarded as the baddie, and we often wish it away. However, the hypodermis provides the primary structural support for the skin. It connects the skin with the bones and muscles, giving you unique facial features.

The fat layer gives form to your face; without it, you would have a ghostly and sunken look. Without the fat layer, humans would look downright scary.

Furthermore, it protects against injuries, promotes skin repair, and regulates hair regeneration speed. It insulates the body from temperature fluctuations. But this fatty layer has one more surprise: It produces leptin, the hormone that tells the body it has had enough to eat! How can we not love fatty hypodermis? It is vital for our looks and nudges us to eat less!

Quick Reminder

cytes: usually used as a suffix, meaning cell

corneocytes: the dead cells on the outermost layer of the skin, consisting primarily of keratin

fibroblasts: cells in the connective tissue of the skin that give structure and produce collagen

keratinocytes: a cell that produces keratin

dendritic: an immune cell

melanocytes: a cell that produces melanin, the colour pigment

matrix cell: a cell that can change from fluid to a gel and back to fluid

mast cell: a cell that releases histamine to fight inflammation

General Terminology

anatomy: how the skin is structured

appendages: down growth from the skin inward during the embryo stage (hair, nails, certain glands, etc.)

cranial nerve: a set of paired nerves at the back of the brain that sends electrical messages

desquamation: a natural process in which the dead cells on the skin are shed to make place for new cells

programmed death: natural death of a cell to make way for a new cell

physiology: the skin's function

squamous: looks like fish scales

glands: an organ that makes substances

apocrine glands: sweat glands in the armpits

eccrine glands: sweat glands on the face

sebaceous gland: a gland that produces sebum in the hair follicle

Substances

collagen: main protein found in the skin

elastin: protein found in the skin, helps skin to stretch and return to its original shape and size

hyaluronic acid: water-binding molecules with an important role in several physiological processes that help with collagen and elastin production

lipids: oils in the skin

fatty acids: a type of lipid

urea: waste product generated by the breakdown of proteins

uric acid: a waste product found in the blood

Chapter 2:
Skin Type and Identification

Everything has beauty, but not everyone sees it.

Sadly, Confucius was right. Many women don't see their own beauty. From early childhood, we are conditioned to compare ourselves to the perfect pictures of celebrities in the media. We forget that these women have make-up teams, hairdressers, and probably personal shoppers who work as a production team to present a professional 'product' to the world.

Moreover, the camera team uses every available technological device to create an artful end product. Ten to one, celebrities look considerably less glorious when they wake up in the morning to the demands of a difficult day.

During the past two decades, social media has become a powerful force and plays a significant role in our social and personal lives. Of course, social media is by no means only negative. On the contrary, it has numerous benefits: It connects us to the world, broadens our horizons, and enriches our personal lives. We build stimulating relationships, share each others' experiences, and gain knowledge via the internet.

Since the beginning of time, appearance has been important, and it still is. Visual communication has always been part of life; many examples exist in animal life. Male birds use their colourful feathers to attract females. Chimpanzees raise their arms and slap the ground to intimidate. The poison dart frog is bright orange, warning predators not to eat them (Khan Academy, n.d.).

Similarly, over the centuries, humans have used visual communication consciously or subconsciously to display status and attractiveness and send non-verbal messages. Generally, good-looking people are rated more successful and popular than their plainer colleagues.

Social media has taken visual communication to a different level, with overemphasis on the outward appearance and not reflecting any of the inner qualities of the personality. Most social media users post selfies portraying themselves in the best light possible. Furthermore, we are constantly confronted by images of beautiful people on our screens.

We know that with smartphone technology, these images are photoshopped into near-perfect images. Still, one's self-esteem might suffer when comparing oneself with perfect images.

In a recent article published in the *European Scientific Journal*, researchers reported that 88% of Facebook users compared themselves with online pictures. Moreover, the researchers found a strong indication that self-esteem decreased with the increase in time spent on Facebook (Jan, 2017).

Back to Confucius' words. You are unique. You must learn to recognise and internalise it. You might not have the type of hair that trends at the moment. You might be overweight or have bad skin. But somewhere there lurks a well-kept and cared-for version of you. Perhaps a visit to a good hairdresser, a dermatologist, and regular walks with the dog are needed to reveal the better-looking you.

Take note: Beauty has different dimensions. Of course, hair, skin, and being well-built contribute to your attractiveness. But being well-cared for and well-kept are important aspects of being attractive, if not beautiful, in conventional terms. It is true for all ages but becomes increasingly important as a woman ages. *A well-kept woman is an attractive woman.*

Here's the dilemma, though: Sometimes life breaks your self-esteem down bit by bit, and you get stuck in the kids' programmes, your partner's lives, and your problems. Your subconscious tells you that your loved ones must come first. In the process, you start neglecting yourself.

Admittedly, it is difficult to feel beautiful if you speed through the days like a bullet train through the Russian steppes. Maybe this is the time for a cliché: You must appreciate yourself and your unique looks to regain self-esteem.

Of course, there will always be a more attractive person than you. Still, deep down, you must remember that your appearance does not determine your value as a human being. Besides, those images you jealously admire are not even authentic.

Recent research reports that self-care and wellness are increasingly regarded as health issues. A healthy lifestyle is vital for a healthy body. A healthy body, again, is a prerequisite for good skin. Appearance has thus become a health issue, and self-care is necessary to look good and be healthy. Fitness, healthy eating, and personal body and skincare are generally accepted as the norm in modern society.

Join this health-is-beauty trend today. You cannot feel beautiful if you are not healthy and well-kept. Does this sound a bit like pie in the sky? Let us then get down to the basics. Start loving yourself with a few minutes here and there. As one of the big names in skincare and cosmetics says so often in their marketing flashes: 'Because you're worth it.'

Your skin is the gift wrapping; you are the real gift. You present yourself to the world wrapped beautifully or carelessly in your skin. Your skin is often the first thing others see and judge you on. Your skin tells the story of how you take care of yourself before you even speak a word.

Look at yourself in the bathroom mirror. Are you satisfied with what you see? You want your special gift wrapping to be of the best quality and to look as good as possible for yourself.

There are different ways to classify skin types, which are not necessarily in opposition. On the contrary, the cosmetic industry is privileged to use medical research to produce skincare based on sound research and medical knowledge. We will discuss the two systems mostly used, the first a medical and the second a cosmetic classification of skin. Several systems have been developed through the decades, and your medical practitioner might use a different one.

The Medical Way – Fitzpatrick Skin Type (FST)

Since 1975, dermatologists and cosmetologists have used the Fitzpatrick Skin Type (FST) system to classify skin types based on their reaction to the sun. It must be stressed that this system does not classify skin types according to ethnic groups. The classification was never based on skin colour or ethnic group but on *how the skin reacts to sunburn.*

Since 1975 doctors have used FST to determine how patients' skin reacts to sunburn. It was done through self-assessment interviews. The results obtained in this method were semi-subjective, as participants had different interpretations of the terminology used in the questionnaires. Scientists and doctors agree that only dermatologists or medical practitioners should do FST classification.

Your skin's reaction to ultraviolet rays of the sun depends on the melanin levels in the keratinocytes. Melanin protects the skin against ultraviolet rays.

Because self-assessment is not always accurate, some dermatologists use an advanced scientific method to measure the melanin in the skin. Reflectance spectrophotometry determines the skin's reaction to the sun based on skin reflectance. Unfortunately, these tests are not yet generally available.

Fitzpatrick Skin Type I to VI

Based on the Fitzpatrick method, six skin types have been identified, each with distinctive trends. Please note that you might not fit precisely into one type only but might be a combination of two types.

Skin cancer is serious; if in doubt, consult a professional if you have anything bothering you. Knowing your FST is vital to understanding your risk of skin cancer and protecting yourself accordingly.

Skin Type 1

- The natural skin colour is extremely fair.
- The natural hair colour is pale blond or red.
- The eye colour is blue, light grey, or light green.
- When exposed to the sun, the skin burns freckles.
- It always burns and never tans.

Skin Type 2

- The natural skin colour is fair.

- The natural hair colour is blond.

- The eye colour is blue, grey, or green.

- When exposed to the sun, the skin usually has freckles, burns, and peels.

- It rarely tans.

Skin Types 1 and 2: What to Know and What to Do

- You will get sun damage from exposure.

- The sun will age your skin.

- You have a high chance of developing melanoma or skin cancer.

- Use sunscreen with a high sun protection factor (SFP), a hat, and sunglasses that block ultraviolet rays.

- Stay out of the sun and in the shade as much as possible and wear protective clothing.

- Check yourself for changes in your skin every month and visit your doctor once a year for a thorough check-up.

Skin Type 3

- The natural skin colour is fair to beige.

- The natural hair colour is dark blond to light brown.

- The eye colour is hazel to light brown.

- When exposed to the sun, the skin sometimes freckles.

- The skin occasionally burns and sometimes tans.

Skin Type 4

- The natural skin colour is light brown and often described as olive.
- The natural hair colour is dark brown.
- The eye colour is dark brown.
- When exposed to the sun, the skin usually does not freckle or burn.
- The skin tans well.

Skin Type 5

- The natural skin colour is dark brown.
- The natural hair colour is dark brown to black.
- The eye colour is dark brown to black.
- When exposed to the sun, the skin rarely develops freckles and does not burn.
- The skin always tans.

Skin Type 6

- The natural skin colour is dark brown.
- The natural hair colour is black.
- The eye colour is brown-black.
- When exposed to the sun, the skin never has freckles and never burns.
- The skin tans darkly.

Skin Types 3, 4, 5, and 6: What to Know and What to Do

- You are still at risk of sun damage and signs of ageing.

- You are at risk of skin cancer, especially if you have used a sunbed for tanning or have had frequent exposure to the sun.

- Many patients with darker skin delay going to their doctor, as they falsely believe darker skin is not at risk of skin cancer. An early diagnosis of melanoma can save your life.

- Use sunscreen with a sun protection factor (SFP) of at least 15, a hat, and sunglasses that block ultraviolet rays.

- Stay out of the sun and in the shade as much as possible.

- Wear protective clothing if you are in the sun for long periods.

- Check your whole body for changes in your skin every month.

- Visit your doctor once a year for a thorough check-up. People with darker skin may get *Acral lentiginous melanoma*. This type of skin cancer appears on a part of the body that was *no*t exposed to the sun. Therefore, these melanomas are often only discovered at a late stage when they are challenging to treat successfully (Hecht, 2019).

The Cosmetic Way – Skin Condition and Needs

Cosmetic scientists approach skincare from a different viewpoint than medical researchers. Cosmetic science wants to enhance your looks while the medical profession addresses health issues. However, a dermatologist is also trained to help you with conditions such as hyperpigmentation, acne, and other conditions. These might not be life-threatening but may have adverse physical and emotional effects. Together, cosmetic and medical sciences can help you care for your skin and maintain good skin quality.

The cosmetic industry has contributed significantly to the public's changing opinion on the necessity of protection against UV radiation and skin cancer. Although skincare products are designed to retain moisture, cosmeceutical experts also emphasise protection against the sun – a double whammy for the skin. Be warned, though, that you cannot rely on skincare products to protect the skin against the sun; sunscreen is a necessity.

Cosmetic products aim to keep the skin well-balanced and healthy; not too dry, not too oily. Moisture is an important deciding factor in skin classification, and cosmetic scientists classify the skin according to its moisture level, sebaceous secretion, and sensitivity (Almarill, n.d.).

Every skin is different, and only when you have determined your skin type can you make informed choices on skincare products and treatments.

The cosmetic industry has identified five skin types, and research focuses on the individual needs of the five skin types.

Cosmetic Industry Skin Types

Normal Skin

Normal skin is anything but normal; it is the ideal skin type, but few women have normal skin. Normal skin is neither dry nor oily. It has an even texture, with no apparent pores or discolouring. The skin appears clear and soft – every woman's dream, but unfortunately, not the reality for most women. Most women struggle with some aspect of their skin.

Sensitive Skin

Sensitive skin is delicate and reacts to environmental stimuli such as the sun, heat, and cold weather. The skin barrier is not strong enough to protect the skin; consequently, the skin is easily irritated. This type of skin often has rashes, infections, or allergic reactions.

Some refer to this skin type as irritated skin. It is extremely dry, feels tight, and is red and itchy.

Dry Skin

Dry skin shares some of the symptoms of sensitive skin. Dry skin might be genetic, but it can also be attributed to hormonal changes.

Often, external factors dehydrate the skin. Air conditioners, hot water, the sun, tanning beds, and long, hot baths or showers cause dehydration. Avoid excessive cold, heat, and air conditioners as much as possible. Harsh ingredients in cleaners, especially soaps and skincare products, also aggravate dryness.

If your skin is dry despite regular moisturising, change your cleanser to a non-foaming one. You will notice an immediate improvement.

Certain medications also cause dry skin, and you should discuss it with your doctor or pharmacist.

Dry skin looks dull and dehydrated with lines but has no visible pores. However, the skin is less elastic and shows early signs of ageing. Regular moisturising will go far to hydrate your skin.

Oily Skin

Oily skin usually has enlarged pores and a slightly greasy surface. Oily skin is often genetic. The sebaceous glands produce excess sebum, a fat that causes a shiny complexion.

People younger than 30 often suffer from oily skin because hormonal imbalances stimulate excess sebum production.

Combination Skin

Combination skin usually has dry and oily areas. The so-called T-zone (forehead, nose and chin) has more sebaceous glands which produce too much sebum. These areas appear shiny with blackheads and visible pores. The skin on the cheeks is normal or dry.

Baumann Skin Type Indicator (BSTI)

Professor Leslie Baumann, a highly respected researcher, published widely on skin types, and many cosmetic companies base their digital diagnosis models on Baumann's research. She is a cosmetic dermatologist and developed a questionnaire to determine skin type at the University of Miami in 2004. This questionnaire is still widely used by researchers, cosmetic houses, medical professionals, beauticians, and individuals.

It is important to remember that *Baumann's system is based on individual skin properties; Fitzpatrick's system is based on the skin's reaction to the sun* and the risk of skin cancer. The two systems do not oppose each other. You have to be familiar with both. Baumann's classification will help you to choose the correct skincare products. Fitzpatrick's classification will help protect your skin against sun damage and the possibility of skin cancer.

Leslie Baumann designed a digital-based questionnaire to assess four main properties of the skin: oily versus dry, sensitive versus resistant, pigmented versus non-pigmented, and wrinkled versus unwrinkled. These four skin types are further described in terms of the skin's properties or barriers to skin health: dehydration, inflammation, pigmentation, and ageing (Baumann, 2008).

Although most of the terminology in Professor Baumann's skin types is self-explanatory, take note of the following:

- Pigmentation indicates that a skin type overproduces melanin and is prone to developing dark patches when exposed to the sun.

- Sensitive indicates that the skin is easily irritated and develops redness, rashes, itching, or burning. The skin barrier is weak and prone to inflammation. Sensory nerves might have slight abnormalities (Rodan, 2014).

- Resistant indicates that the skin barrier is strong and the skin is resistant to irritants.

Professor Baumann developed 16 sub-categories based on the four main skin types. Study these skin types carefully before you decide on yours. Your skin type will determine which products to buy and which treatments to use. An accurate diagnosis is vital for treating your skin correctly and improving its quality.

Baumanns 16 Skin Types

Oily Sensitive Pigmented Wrinkled (OSPW)

- It does not have problems with dryness as it produces enough sebum.

- It has an uneven tone.

- It shows redness and flushing.

- It has acne breakouts.

- It has rashes and irritation.

- It is prone to inflammation that leads to the darkening of the infected areas.

- It has dark marks (melasma) and freckles.

- It is often red and irritated.

- It wrinkles early.

- Use products that will calm inflammation and stay away from products that will clog pores.

- Use foaming cleansers, retinol, and sunscreen.

- Avoid sun damage and smoking.

Oily Sensitive Pigmented Tight (OSPT)

- Younger people with darker skin and light-skinned *pregnant* women often have this skin type.

- It shines for about an hour after washing the face.

- It shows redness and flushing.

- It has acne breakouts, rashes, and irritation.

- It is prone to inflammation and darkening of areas affected by pimples.

- It often has melasma and freckles.

- It is less prone to wrinkles.

- Wear sunscreen that will not add to the oiliness.

- Choose a cleanser based on your type of sensitivity, acne, redness, or allergies.

- Avoid sun damage and smoking.

Oily Sensitive Non-Pigmented Wrinkled (OSNW)

- It is a very common skin type.

- It shows redness and flushing and is shiny.

- It has intermittent acne breakouts, rashes, and irritation.

- It does not have high pigmentation protection and wrinkles show early.

- It might take a complex skincare routine to address all the problems.

- Use products that contain retinoids.

- This skin often needs an antioxidant supplement.

- Use sunscreen with an SPF of at least 15.

- Avoid sun damage and smoking.

- See a dermatologist if you have persistent skin irritations or conditions.

Oily Sensitive Non-Pigmented Tight (OSNT)

- It has redness, rashes, and irritation and a high risk for rosacea.

- It has intermittent acne breakouts, pimples, and bumps with a dent in the middle.

- It has visible red or blue blood vessels on the face.

- It is non-pigmented.

- It does not wrinkle early because of its pigmentation protection.

- It improves with ageing, as the skin becomes dryer.

- Use anti-inflammation products.

- Avoid sun damage and smoking.

Oily Resistant Pigmented Wrinkled (ORPW)

- This skin type can improve when treated with the right products from a young age.

- It soon shows signs of ageing and has large pores.

- It has acne breakouts.

- It has redness and skin rashes.

- It has dark patches (melasma) and freckles.

- Use skin products with high concentrations of active ingredients to combat wrinkles.

- Avoid stress, get adequate sleep, and follow a healthy diet.

- Use skincare products with retinoids and vitamin C.

- Avoid sun damage and smoking.

- Follow a healthy lifestyle to improve typical ORPW problems.

Oily Resistant Pigmentation Tight (ORPT)

- It rarely has acne breakouts, redness, or rashes.
- It is prone to hyperpigmentation and scarring.
- It has dark patches (melasma) and freckles.
- It does not wrinkle early because of its natural sebum production.
- Always wear sunscreen with a high SPF.
- Follow a healthy lifestyle.

Oily Resistant Non-Pigmentation Wrinkled (ORNW)

- It soon shows signs of ageing.
- It rarely has acne breakouts, redness, or rashes.
- It does not have high pigmentation protection and wrinkles show early.
- Use products that combat oiliness and prevent wrinkles.
- Avoid sun damage and smoking.
- It has a strong protective skin barrier.

Oily Resistant Non-Pigmentation Tight (ORNT)

- It is the ideal skin type.
- It rarely has acne breakouts, redness, or rashes.
- It does not wrinkle early because of its pigmentation protection.
- Use products that combat oiliness but do not harm the skin's natural sebum.
- Follow a healthy lifestyle.

Dry Sensitive Pigmented Wrinkled (DSPW)

- It is a challenging skin type and often needs medical attention.

- Your skin might not fit 100% into the DSPW description. Consult a professional if you experience problems.

- Individual analysis and treatment might be necessary.

- It is prone to dehydration as its sebum production decreases with age.

- It looks rough.

- It ages quickly.

- Some anti-ageing products and skin-lightening products can be harmful.

- It has acne breakouts.

- It has redness, rashes, and flushes.

- It has inflammation and develops dark patches (melasma) and freckles.

- The skin barrier is weak, and consequently, it is prone to dehydration and dark spots.

- Use an oil, cream, or milk-based cleanser.

- Use anti-inflammatory ingredients.

- Avoid toners that contain alcohol.

- Use sunscreens with an oil base.

- Avoid mechanical exfoliation such as scrubs and microdermabrasion.

- Follow a healthy lifestyle, get adequate sleep, and do not smoke.

Dry Sensitive Pigmentation Tight (DSPT)

- It can be improved with daily and appropriate skincare.

- Many people with a medium skin tone have DSPT.

- It often looks ashen with an uneven tone.

- It has acne breakouts.

- It has rashes and irritations, even eczema.

- The skin barrier is weak and, consequently, it is prone to dehydration and dark spots.

- Use a creamy cleanser that does not strip your skin of oil.

- Use moisturisers that target barrier repair.

- Always use sunscreen.

- Follow a healthy lifestyle.

Dry Sensitive Non-Pigmentation Wrinkled (DSNW)

- It is a complex skin and must be treated according to its specific problem.

- It has acne breakouts.

- It has rashes and redness.

- The skin barrier is weak and, consequently, it is prone to dehydration and skin rashes.

- It wrinkles early and quickly.

- Use products with anti-inflammatory ingredients and take anti-inflammatory supplements.

- Use barrier repair moisturisers and do not take retinoids every day.

- Do not use toners that contain alcohol, as it dries your skin.

- Always use sunscreen.

- Follow a healthy lifestyle and work on your stress levels.

Dry Sensitive Pigmentation Wrinkled (DSPW)

- It is a challenging skin type and often needs medical attention, as it does not necessarily fit into the general DSPW type.

- It is prone to skin cancer and must be checked regularly.

- It does not produce enough sebum and is dehydrated.

- It appears rough and lacks radiance.

- It has acne breakouts.

- It has rashes and redness.

- The skin barrier is weak and consequently, it is prone to dehydration and skin rashes.

- Use cream-based cleansers.

- Use products with anti-inflammatory ingredients and use anti-inflammatory supplements.

- Use barrier repair moisturisers.

- Do not use toners that contain alcohol, as it dries the skin.

- Always use sunscreen with a built-in moisturiser.

- Follow a healthy lifestyle.

Dry Resistant Pigmentation Wrinkled (DRPW)

- It has acne breakouts.

- It has rashes and redness.

- It has melanin that can develop pigmentation, dark patches (melasma), and freckles.

- Look for skin products designed to help with pigmentation.

- Do not use too many products together, as their active ingredients can clash.

- It has a strong protective skin barrier but still tends to develop wrinkles.

- Follow a healthy lifestyle and avoid the sun.

Dry Resistant Pigmentation Tight (DRPT)

- It has an uneven skin tone.

- It has acne breakouts.

- It has rashes and redness.

- It has melanin that can cause pigmentation and dark spots, especially after an injury.

- The skin barrier is weak and does not retain water.

- Cleanse with cream-based products.

- Use a barrier repair moisturiser.

- It has a lower tendency to wrinkle.

- Use sunscreen with at least an SPF of 15.

- Do not take very hot baths or showers.

- Follow a healthy lifestyle.

- Look for skin products designed to help with pigmentation.

Dry Resistant Non-Pigmentation Wrinkled (DRNW)

- Ageing skin commonly falls into this skin category.

- It has acne breakouts.

- It has rashes and redness.

- It does not have enough pigmentation protection.

- It tends to wrinkle.

- Avoid soap.

- Follow a healthy lifestyle.

- Avoid the sun and always wear sunscreen of at least 30 SPF.

Dry Resistant Non-Pigmentation Tight (DRNT)

- It rarely has acne breakouts, redness, or rashes.

- The skin has rough patches, uneven cells, and skin tone.

- It does not have enough pigmentation protection.

- It is slow to sag and also slow to form wrinkles.

- It has a strong protective skin barrier; thus, this skin needs products with active ingredients, such as retinol.

- Use a fragrance-free moisturiser.

- Follow a healthy lifestyle.

- Avoid the sun and smoking.

The next chapter discusses skincare products and their key ingredients in more detail. Before deciding on what products or treatments to buy, it is essential to know your skin type.

Quick Reminder

Acceptance and Commitment Therapy (ACT): accepting negative thoughts and emotions; let them go and return to your core values and beliefs

Baumann Skin Type Indicators (BSTI): a digital-based questionnaire based on four properties of the skin and the various combinations between them: oily versus dry, sensitive versus resistant, pigmented versus non-pigmented, and wrinkled versus unwrinkled

Fitzpatrick Skin Type (FST): classifies skin types based on their reaction to the sun and their tendency to get skin cancer

Reflectance Spectrophotometry: measuring the skin's reaction to the sun based on skin reflectance and the amount of melanin in the keratinocytes

reflectance: visible light reflected by the skin surface

spectrophotometry: determines the relation between the reflected light of the skin surface and the amount of melanin in the keratinocytes

Sun Protection Factor (SPF): measures how much UV radiation (sunlight) will be needed to burn the skin when the skin is protected; the more protection the skin needs, the higher the SPF should be pigmentation: indicates that the skin overproduces melanin and, consequently, is prone to develop dark patches when exposed to the sun

sensitive: suggests that the skin is easily irritated and develops redness, rashes, itching, or burning

resistant: indicates that the skin barrier is strong and the skin is resistant to irritants

Chapter 3:
Skincare Products and Ingredients

Beauty awakens the soul to act.

The works of Dante Alighieri, better known as Dante and arguably the most enduring poet of all time, have survived since the 13th century and could hardly be improved. He might not have had skincare in mind when he said, 'Knowledge about your individual beauty awakens you to act,' but it is excellent advice for women in the 21st century.

In the previous chapter, individual skin types were discussed. You owe it to yourself to take the Fitzpatrick system very seriously. Prevention is better than cure, especially when it comes to skin cancer. You also owe it to yourself to study the Baumann system to ensure you use the most effective ingredients. The wrong products can be wasted on your skin and can even do some harm. Do not waste money and miss the opportunity to make the most of your skin by using the wrong products.

The cosmetic industry is extensive, and consumers are often confused by the endless number of available products. Highly effective marketing is vital in any competitive sector to reach potential clients. Aggressive marketing slogans are not designed to educate you but to convince you to buy a specific product. The advertised product might not even be suitable for your skin type. You are not alone if, sometimes, you are overwhelmed by all the excellent (and not-so-good) products and their marketing promises.

Knowledge of skincare and skincare products will save you money and improve your skin quality considerably. Do not rely on advertisements, shop assistants, friends, or colleagues for advice. Do your research, determine your skin type, and study the following sections for the best ingredients for your skin. It is of utmost importance that you know your skin type and the best skincare ingredients for its specific needs.

Skincare Programme

This chapter will not concentrate on the different skincare steps or the variety of products available for each step. It gives information on the ingredients and what they can or cannot do for your skin.

This guide is not about any specific brand or product but the *ingredients*. This chapter gives special attention to the role these ingredients play in keeping your skin healthy and fresh. Use your knowledge, find independent reviews, and analyse the ingredient list before buying. If samples are available, test them before you buy them. Skincare is expensive, and you must make an informed choice for the sake of your skin and pocket.

Skincare ingredients can be confusing. Therefore, it is good to understand what they mean, how they work, and why they are used together.

Don't let scientific names and, especially, the abbreviations confuse you. The cosmetic industry uses abbreviations presumably because the name of a single ingredient often consists of two or even three words. In this chapter, we give both the full name and the abbreviation. At the cost of sounding repetitive, the full name of an ingredient is used to prevent confusion.

Terminology in Skincare Explained

Active Ingredients

Active ingredients in a skincare product do precisely as their name says. They act on your skin. They target specific problems such as acne, fine lines, or hyperpigmentation. Cosmetic scientists researched and formulated products with active ingredients to address a particular skin condition.

Often, active ingredients do not work on their own. Think of a teabag and boiling water; you can't make tea without the water. Usually, a few ingredients are specifically included to prompt the active ingredient to do its work.

In the following section of this chapter, several of these active ingredients are discussed: alpha-hydroxy acids (AHAs), hyaluronic acid (HA), vitamin C, vitamin A or retinol, and SPF (Mehra, 2021).

Your products usually have several ingredients. Most are water- or oil-based and have a particular function. However, all of them work together for maximum effect on your skin.

Acids

Many people associate acids with harmful substances, which are dangerous and scary. Quite the contrary, the stratum corneum is naturally slightly acidic, and the acidity level needs to be maintained. The natural skin acids help keep the keratinocytes (the protein cells) tightly bound. This near-solid skin barrier protects the skin and prevents water loss.

The skin's natural acidity varies between pH4,5 and 6,5. Anything higher causes the skin to be too alkaline. Soaps, for example, are alkaline and dehydrate the skin (Cherney, 2019).

Alpha-hydroxy and hyaluronic acids are discussed later in this chapter, as they are popular ingredients in skincare.

Allergens

An allergen is a substance that potentially may cause an allergic reaction. A healthy person's immune system usually reacts when allergens are detected. It produces an antibody that prevents the allergen from harming the skin. When the immune system is compromised, allergens can cause skin problems.

There are many common allergens: animal proteins, dust, fungal spores, insect bites and faeces, mite faeces, and pollen. Some prescription medicines might also cause allergic reactions, as do some foods (MedlinePlus, n.d.).

Free Radicals

Free radicals are molecules derived from oxygen and are known as reactive oxygen species (ROS). Very importantly, they have an uneven number of electrons. Because the electrons are not evenly balanced, they have to bind with other molecules to stabilise: this process damages skin cells, fatty tissue, proteins, and DNA.

Remember, you are naturally exposed to free radicals every day. They are all around us. The ozone layer contains free radicals because of smoking, pesticides, chemical products, and environmental pollution. Your diet might add to free radicals in the body. In Chapter 10, the effects of sugar, fat, and alcohol on free radicals is discussed.

Antioxidants neutralise free radicals because they can provide the missing electron. The free radical is thus stabilised without any harm done.

Antioxidants

Antioxidants are invaluable in preventing the damage free radicals can do to skin cells. Antioxidants come mostly from plants. Vegetables and fruits have plenty of natural antioxidants, especially berries, cherries, citrus, prunes, dark leafy greens, broccoli, carrots, tomatoes, and olives. Vitamins, fish, and nuts are also natural sources of antioxidants.

Vitamins contain antioxidants and are often used in skincare products. However, several other antioxidants protect the skin barrier from negative environmental effects and can reverse signs of ageing.

Nonetheless, a healthy lifestyle is the best for cultivating antioxidants. Exercise, sleep, limited alcohol consumption, and a healthy diet provide antioxidants to the body. Avoid smoking and pollution at all costs; they destroy antioxidants.

Pathogens

A pathogen is a medical term for a bacterium, virus, or microorganism that can cause disease. In general terms, skin pathogens are infections.

Emollients, Occlusives, and Humectants

Terminology can be confusing, and deciphering labels is a nightmare. Emollients, humectants, and occlusives sometimes overlap. A specific skincare ingredient can simultaneously be an emollient, occlusive, and/or a humectant. In this guide, they are discussed separately, as each has particular properties. What is essential is that all three are moisturisers.

- **Emollients**

Emollients are moisturisers and, like all moisturisers, form a layer on the skin which traps moisture and soothes the skin. Skincare emollients come in different formulas; lotions, creams, and ointments. Emollients fill the tiny spaces around the dead cells, and the skin appears smoother in texture.

Look out for the following emollients on labels: lanolin, beeswax, mineral oil, petroleum, shea butter, and safflower oil. Emollients are sometimes listed as lipids, oils, silicones, or barrier repair.

- **Humectants**

Humectants attract water from the air and bind with water already in the skin. They are stalwarts in many skincare and haircare products.

Humectants might even go beyond retaining water in the skin. It is speculated that some humectants break down the dead cells on the stratum corneum. The dead cells cause a rough and uneven skin tone. Skin shedding, or desquamation, occurs when the stratum corneum's water content is below 10% (WebMD, 2021). Furthermore, some experts say humectants draw water from the deeper layers of the skin.

For humectants to function correctly, they must stay on the skin. Therefore, they are often combined with occlusives to remain intact on the skin surface.

Some of the best-known humectants – hyaluronic acid, glycerin, and alpha-hydroxy acids – are discussed in more detail in the section on ingredients.

- **Occlusives**

Your grandmother was right all the time: Lanolin is a reliable moisturiser and occlusive. It is obtained from sheep sebaceous glands and can reduce water loss by 20 to 30% (Purnamawati, 2017).

Occlusives are vital for retaining moisture from evaporation and are invaluable in keeping your skin hydrated. They also prevent pathogens and irritants from penetrating and harming the skin.

Occlusives are instrumental in keeping humectants stuck on the skin surface. Occlusives, emollients, and humectants work together to moisturise and protect your skin. Humectants bind with water, and occlusives and emollients stop evaporation and thus retain moisture in the stratum corneum (Wizemann, 2020).

Occlusives and emollients are often found in the same products: petroleum, lanolin, silicones, carnauba wax, beeswax, shea butter, castor oil, and a variety of other plant butters and oils. If your skin is dry, use a product with occlusives.

Safe Preservatives

Consumers are very aware of chemicals and understandably hesitant about the preservatives in their products. Unfortunately, chemical preservatives are necessary to preserve a product and keep it fresh and intact.

Without preservatives, bacteria and other harmful substances will spoil your expensive products within days and might even harm your skin.

Preservatives should be non-toxic and non-irritating to the skin. Unfortunately, many preservatives and fragrances have the opposite effect and cause allergies. Especially if your skin is sensitive, you should investigate the preservative list in the product. Alternatively, patch test a new product before buying to see how your skin will react.

Do not use products with harmful preservatives such as parabens and formaldehyde. Parabens can potentially mimic oestrogen and increase the risk of breast cancer.

We all know that formaldehyde was used in ancient times to embalm bodies, proof that it is an excellent preservative. However, it can cause several illnesses, including leukaemia and brain cancer.

There are several safe preservatives. Make sure that your skincare products contain safe preservatives. If you are in doubt, consult your doctor or pharmacist.

Solvents

Skincare solvents are liquids such as water, vegetable oil, animal oils, silicones, and alcohol. You will find solvents in nail varnish remover, mouthwash, toothpaste, lotions, creams, and most hair products.

Key ingredients sometimes need to be combined with a solvent for easier application; thus, solvents are essential for most skincare products.

Skincare Ingredients Explained

Alpha-Hydroxy Acids (AHAs)

We often hear about alpha-hydroxy acids and see them mentioned in marketing material and ingredient lists. Several animal- and plant-based alpha-hydroxy acids are often used as active ingredients in skincare. Some of these alpha-hydroxy acids we know from cooking are citric acid (citrus foods), lactic acid (lactose), and tartaric acid (grapes).

Lactic acids are regularly used in cosmetics. Another common acid in skincare is glycolic acid, which should not be confused with glycerin. Glycolic acid is found in sugar cane and grapes. Glycolic acid is the simplest of alpha-hydroxy acids. Its small organic oil molecules contain both alcohol and acidic components. It has few salts and is water-soluble, making it easy to remove.

Primarily, alpha-hydroxy acids are excellent for exfoliating the dead cells from the stratum corneum. Although the skin gets rid of dead cells through desquamation, the rate at which cells are shed decreases with age. Dead cells cause rough and uneven skin tone, every woman's nightmare. Alpha-hydroxy acids speed up the shedding of dead cells and make way for new cells, visibly improving skin complexion.

But alpha-hydroxy acids in skincare have many other uses: treatment of pigmentation, prevention of acne, and improvement of the complexion and fine wrinkles. Last but not least, it promotes collagen production.

Glycerin

Glycerin is not related to glycolic acid and is also not an alpha-hydroxy acid.

It is a byproduct of biodiesel production and is also found in animal and plant sources. Pure glycerin (glycerol) is alcohol. Glycerine is the commercial version and is used very successfully in skincare.

It has quite a scary history, though. In the 1800s, dynamite was made with glycerin (Petre, 2018). Fortunately, we and glycerin have come a long way, and glycerin today forms an essential ingredient in cosmetics.

Although pure glycerin might cause blisters, glycerin in diluted form often forms the base ingredient for a range of skincare products and soaps. It is odourless and non-toxic. Glycerin dissolves in water and alcohol but not oil.

Rich vegetable fats such as palm, soy, and coconut oil are heated to separate the glycerin from the natural fatty acids. Some studies have shown that glycerin products improved hydration in as little as ten days (Petre, 2019).

Hyaluronic Acid (HA)

Although the names sound vaguely the same, hyaluronic acid is also not part of the alpha-hydroxy acid group. Where alpha-hydroxy acids strip the dead layers of the topmost layer of the epidermis, hyaluronic acid is a moisturiser.

The skin gradually produces less hyaluronic acid as we age, and our skin gets drier. The fibroblasts and keratinocytes in the dermis produce hyaluronic acid. Some hyaluronic acid is also found in the epicellular spaces of the spinous layer in the lower parts of the epidermis.

Hyaluronic acid has the remarkable ability to bind with water – up to 1,000 times its weight in water (Baumann, 2014). It is thus also a humectant (see above). Most cosmetic houses use hyaluronic acid in their products, but not all the claims on their labels have been scientifically proven.

Some cosmetic companies want you to believe that the stratum corneum absorbs hyaluronic acid. Several dermatologists oppose this claim quite strongly. They say hyaluronic acid cannot penetrate the hard stratum corneum to reach the lower layers of the skin (Baumann, 2014).

Should we then even use products containing hyaluronic acid? Is it even a moisturiser? The answer is: Yes. Even if the stratum corneum cannot absorb it, surface hyaluronic acid is a humectant and binds with water. Consequently, it retains moisture and keeps the skin surface hydrated (F.C. Simple Skincare Science, 2019).

Transepidermal water loss (TEWL) measures how much water evaporates from your skin. A moisturiser containing hyaluronic acid forms a layer on the stratum corneum and prevents your skin's natural moisture from evaporating. Hyaluronic acid's ability to bind with water thus plays a vital role in retaining water in the skin.

Ceramides

Ceramides are oils in your skin and the skin's natural moisturisers. They also protect the skin from external germs as they form a shield on the surface. Ceramides are a chain of carbon atoms with amino acids attached. These chains allow ceramides to bind with other fatty acids, a valuable ally in strengthening the skin barrier.

There are 12 types of ceramides. Like all the cells in the skin, ceramides decrease as you grow older, and your skin will get drier. Researchers found that the levels of ceramide types 1 to 6 decrease in ageing skin (Kunde, 2021).

The good news is that you can apply topical ceramides successfully, as they are present in the stratum corneum. Topical ceramides can thus supplement the skin's natural ceramides. You might be surprised to hear that most ceramides in skincare are synthetic. Synthetic ceramides are free of contamination, and therefore safe to use.

Collagen and Peptides, Topical Application, and Supplements

Collagen

Topically applied collagen moisturises the skin but is too large to penetrate the skin. Natural collagen is undeniably the main structural component of the skin and is primarily produced and found in the dermis. It forms a fibrous protein structure with elastin to support the skin.

The natural collagen molecules in your body are very hard and, gram for gram, stronger than steel.

Collagen forms between 25 to 35% of your body, and 29 types of collagen are known to researchers. Type 1 is found in the skin. It strengthens the skin, helps with elasticity, and removes dead skin cells. Unfortunately, adults' collagen production decreases by about 1% each year. This leads to a loss of firmness (Krant, 2017).

It has not been proven that the much smaller collagen peptides (see below) can penetrate the skin and stimulate collagen production. Fortunately, there are several natural ways to stimulate collagen production. Both oral intake and topical application of vitamin C improve collagen production. The topical application of retinoids, specifically the synthetic form tretinoin, is also very effective.

Peptides

Peptides are often referred to as collagen-peptides. They are not the same as collagen proteins, though. Peptides are short chains of amino acids which combine to form collagen, keratin, and elastin, the body's main building blocks.

Peptides and vitamin A derivatives (retinol) are cell regulators, as they directly influence collagen production.

Although there are conflicting schools of thought on how and whether peptides are effective, peptides seem to slow down ageing. Collagen peptide supplements and topically applied peptides have been on the market for some time. Many users are convinced both supplements and topical peptides improve the skin, nails, and hair. Medical professionals and journalists are still hesitant to support these claims openly. They are careful in their reports and use terms such as 'might help' or 'could have helped'.

Studies must involve significant numbers of participants to obtain credible results. Furthermore, scientific reports have to be accepted by peers in the field. Research is costly, and researchers often prefer not to be sponsored by a specific company. They want their findings to be impartial and not under suspicion of being biassed.

Unfortunately, despite numerous positive reports from consumers, cosmetic companies cannot with certainty state that their collagen peptide products work for the skin. An interesting theory holds that peptides are so small that the body can absorb them. It means that they could potentially enter the lower layers of the skin and eventually the bloodstream and intestines.

Another exciting theory is that, when applied topically, signal peptides might prompt the skin to produce collagen (E Medical, 2017). Still, advocates of signal peptides admit that their claims are not yet scientifically proven.

There are two peptide supplement types: collagen peptides (aimed at skin health and anti-ageing) and keratin peptides (aimed at building strength and muscles). Despite scientific shortcomings, they are popular.

Natural sources of collagen are eggs, milk, meat, fish, shellfish, pulses, oats, and a variety of seeds, wheat, and soybeans. Try peptides if you are desperate to improve your skin, nails, and hair and can afford them. Researchers report that adverse side effects are unlikely (Leonard, 2019).

Elastin

Elastin allows the skin to stretch and return to its normal condition. This protein is found in elastic fibres and is vital for the skin structure. Elastin formation starts in the womb and occurs in the skin, lungs, and blood vessels.

It forms part of the skin structure as its fibres run perpendicular to the skin surface, contributing to its strength and elasticity.

With age, the elastic fibres degrade. Unfortunately, external factors contribute to this process. The sun affects elastin fibres in the epidermis junction (the membrane connecting the epidermis and the dermis). UV radiation (sunburn) has detrimental effects on nearly every part of the human skin, and over-exposure might be the worst thing we can do to our skin.

Elastin has a low turnover rate, and UV radiation harms elastin in two ways: The fibres are shortened, and the protein is also damaged. The ideal would be to replenish the skin's elasticity through topical lotions or supplements. Unfortunately, no scientifically backed treatment to replace elastin is available.

Eating a healthy diet, staying out of the sun, keeping the skin hydrated, and regularly using retinoids can prevent the rapid degeneration of elastin fibres. At present, there is no topical lotion or supplement that can restore your skin's natural elastin.

Petroleum

Who is not familiar with the good old petroleum jelly we used for scratches as kids? It has been with us since the 1950s, when chemist Robert Cheseborough first used the thick gel found on oil wells. Petroleum has been announced safe by the Canadian Cosmetic, Toiletry, and Fragrance Association, but other authorities warn against possible contamination by cancer-causing chemicals found in crude oil. Just for the record: It is rated as moderately unsafe (Best Health, 2022).

Many companies got on the 'petroleum-free' bandwagon and found other moisturiser alternatives. Others believe that the petroleum in skincare is highly refined and meets the standards set by the Canadian cosmetic authority.

Petroleum excellently seals off the skin, retains its moisture, and contributes to skin healing. Some dermatologists go so far as to say it's the most effective moisturiser (Best Health, 2022). Prominent British dermatologists agree that it is safe, and the American Academy of Dermatology recommends petroleum jelly for diaper rash, eczema, and dehydrated skin (Summers, 2022).

Vitamin A (Retinoids/Retinol/Retin-A)

Retinoids form part of a group of compounds derived from vitamin A. Retin-A is the retail name for the drug *tretinoin*, a synthetic version of vitamin A. Retin-A is much stronger than the natural retinol (Palmer, 2020).

Retinoids are cell regulators, as they directly influence collagen production. Consequently, they are trusted stalwarts in skincare, and most modern skincare products contain retinol. It is often used to treat acne, for skin-brightening, and in anti-wrinkle treatments. It stimulates new collagen cell growth in the dermis, and there is growing evidence that retinoids also improve elasticity.

One cannot but be amazed by the complexity of the human skin. For instance, retinol must be converted into retinoic acid before it becomes active in the skin. This process does not happen at the same tempo in everyone and depends on the retinol concentration and the presence of specific enzymes in the skin.

Moreover, the conversion of retinol to retinoic acid is a slow process. Therefore, you have to be patient when using retinol products. It can take six months to see a change (Palmer, 2020).

Remember to take extra precautions when using retinol, as your skin will be more susceptible to UV radiation. You must wear sunscreen to prevent pigmentation. The retinol in your product is not always listed as retinol; thus, make sure when you are in doubt. The higher retinol is listed on the label, the stronger the concentration is.

If you are confused about which ingredient to use, apply vitamins in the morning and acids at night (Mehra, 2021).

Vitamin B3 (Niacin)

Niacin is a nutrient with many functions in the body. It helps lower cholesterol, relieves arthritis pain, and stimulates brain function. Furthermore, it acts as a signal to repair DNA and is an antioxidant.

It can be taken as a supplement in beef, liver, poultry, eggs, fish, nuts, seeds, legumes, avocados, and whole grains. In other words, if you eat healthily, your body and skin have access to natural sources of vitamin B3.

Vitamin C

We have known vitamin C from our earliest childhood days. We loved orange juice for its freshness, and our mothers loved its health benefits. Vitamin C can be taken orally and as a topical treatment. It helps brighten the skin, stimulates collagen production, and lightens pigmentation marks.

A great all-rounder when it comes to achieving brighter, healthier-looking skin, vitamin C delivers in three key areas: stimulating collagen production, fading hyperpigmentation, and reversing the signs of UV damage. It speeds up your skin's natural renewal process, reduces the signs of past damage, and prevents further damage. It also protects against free radicals such as UV rays and pollution.

Vitamin E

Vitamin E has been a buzzword in skincare for many years. But what does it do for your skin? As with the majority of ingredients in skincare, vitamin E is predominantly a moisturiser that seals water in the skin and, in doing so, hydrates the skin. It is a powerful antioxidant that fights free radicals.

But the best news is still to come. It is not proven beyond all doubt, but some studies found that vitamin E might absorb the UVB rays and thus lessen sun damage. However, it is important not to rely on vitamin E for sun protection. Vitamin E does not protect against UV type A radiation.

It might also reduce inflammation of the skin. You can apply vitamin E to the skin to protect the epidermis's top and middle layers.

It dissolves in fat and occurs naturally in the body's sebum. We know that sebum forms a natural barrier to protect the skin. If you have oily skin and suffer from acne, your skin probably already has enough vitamin E.

Once again, a healthy diet should provide you with enough natural vitamin E. Eat broccoli, spinach, kiwi, mango, nuts, and seed oils. Vitamin E is also available in supplements. Just remember, vitamin E is not a magic potion. You won't see a difference overnight. You have to stick to a programme of healthy living and skincare to enhance your skin quality.

Stem Cells

Research into wound healing has opened the door for stem cells to be used in skincare products, another example of how cosmeceutical companies benefit from medical research.

Presently, most products on the market contain an extract from plant stem cells. Cosmeceutical researchers believe stem cells can penetrate the skin much deeper than most other ingredients. Therefore, they work at a deep cellular level to treat wrinkles, accelerate cell turnover, and improve skin texture and tone. Stem cells have protein, peptides, and amino acids – the body's natural building blocks for repairing old cells and building new ones. They also have antioxidant properties, and thus fight free radicals.

Cosmeceutical companies prefer to use plant stem cells over human cells to prevent transmitting any diseases. More research is necessary to use stem cells from animals and humans.

However, human stem cells have unique abilities. They have the amazing ability to replace other cell types and even take over their functions. Furthermore, they signal body cell regeneration; can divide and even repair damaged tissue.

Quick Reminder

Skincare products do not penetrate the skin, not even the dry skin barrier of the stratum corneum.

Skincare products' greatest value is forming a protective layer that keeps natural moisture in the skin.

Even though skincare cannot reach the deeper layers of the skin, the right product is necessary to maximise your natural skin type. Therefore it is vital to know your skin type and choose the right products.

Do not expect immediate miracles. All products take time to work, and you should use small quantities at a time.

Stay out of the sun; it might be the biggest factor in anti-ageing skincare.

Chapter 4:
Ethnic and Unique Beauty

In diversity is beauty.

Mary Angelou died in 2014, but her poems, essays, and memories still radiate the wisdom this remarkable poet left us.

If only women could believe Angelou's words – not only superficially but take them as their motto and believe themselves to be beautiful. Unfortunately for many women, this is not the case. Most women struggle to accept themselves purely because something in their appearance – features, hair, build, or skin colour – does not fit the current fashion trend.

Until about a few decades ago, the ideal beauty was tall, slim, blond, and white. Ironically, very few women fell into this category, and they dyed their hair, wore high heels, followed extreme diets, and even used damaging products to lighten their skin.

Then came social media, which opened the world to millions of women. Social media played a significant role in changing perceptions about beauty. Fuller models started to appear on the billboards, darker skin glowed healthily from our screens, and mesmerising hairstyles challenged the straight and fine blond hairdos.

With the 21st century, beauty in diversity has arrived. But have you accepted your unique body, skin, and appearance as beautiful? Are you still trying to look different and spending loads of money on products that promise to change you to whatever the ideal woman should look like?

The journalist and author Natalie Morris wrote about this dilemma in a heartbreakingly honest article in 2021. She believes TV shows like *The Kardashians* contributed to the changing perception of beauty in the 21st century (Morris, 2021). Suddenly thin, blond models plumbed their lips. Worldwide, big butts became trendy and braids appeared everywhere.

Trends Come and Go

The changing perception of beauty was 'one giant leap for mankind', to borrow from Neil Armstrong.

Beauty is diverse, and your uniqueness is precious. However, there is a but: Do not ride this new beauty wave mindlessly. Don't let the trend of the moment decide your self-esteem. What is fashionable today is out tomorrow. Kick trendy ideas about beauty out and accept, know, and take care of yourself.

Work with what you have. Believe deep down in your core that you are beautiful. Remember, your skin is your gift wrapping, and you are a gift to your loved ones, your friends, colleagues, the world, and yourself. Accept that you are beautiful just as you are, not because it is the current trend. Make the most of yourself, and *never ever* feel the value of your looks depends on a movement.

During the past decade, the beauty world has exploded with skincare products to celebrate the diversity in beauty. Companies now provide unique ranges for a variety of ethnic skin types. The beauty world has finally realised that each ethnic skin type has strong and weak points. Not all fair-skinned women have dry skin, and not all olive-skinned women are guaranteed to tan without sun damage.

Skin Lighteners

Skin lightening creams are available at every supermarket beauty counter and every pharmacy. Many women want a lighter skin tone, and the decision is yours; only you can make the final call.

Lightening creams pose a safety risk. In 2017, the British Skin Foundation reported that 16% of dermatologists rate lightening creams as unsafe, while 80% believe lightening creams should only be used if prescribed by a dermatologist (Malik, 2018). Of course, lightening creams are valuable when treating hyperpigmentation, and in the next chapter, you will learn details about them.

Sadly, many users decide on lightening creams because of the cultural conception that light skin is more attractive. Within some Asian cultures, a lighter skin tone is a status symbol. It can even help you to make a better marriage. Fortunately, the reality of dark-skinned beauty is finally kicking in, and some marriage websites don't allow skin colour to be used as a parameter any longer (Pandey, 2020).

Terminology and Skin Colour

Beauty terminology around ethnicity and race is not clearly defined, and the terms might seem interchangeable. However, there are subtle differences when it comes to skincare. 'Ethnic' usually includes a broader group than race. Because the world has become a global village, people are no longer confined to a specific geographical area. As we migrated across continents and intermarried, new ethnic skin types were formed, and new definitions of skin types were formulated. Women do not fit into narrow racial categories anymore.

In Chapter 2, we discussed Fitzparick's classification, which researchers based on the skin's reaction to sun damage. We also learned about the 16 skin types Professor Leslie Baumann identified. Your race is no longer the deciding factor in skincare; rather, the individual characteristics of your skin within the broader group of skin colours.

In the following sections, you will find information on the good and weak points of the different ethnic categories. These types are not in opposition to Fitzpatrick's or Baumann's systems.

Please remember that the categories discussed here are very broad, and each includes millions of women. This section discusses the advantages and disadvantages in general categories. For detailed information on your skin type, consult the Fitzpatrick and Baumann classification systems.

This chapter aims to convince you that your skin colour matters, *not your race*. Moreover, skin colour is genetic, and your genes determine whether you are prone to specific skin problems. This chapter informs you about your skin's potential issues but also about your skin's strong points. Just like life, your skin type has benefits and also drawbacks.

Many of the most common skin problems occur in all ethnic groups but might be more prominent in one skin colour. It is thus wise to check with the information in this chapter's sections.

Melanin, Skin Colour, and Sun Damage

Melanin is a pigment found in the hair, skin, and iris, and it determines your hair, eye, and skin colour. But it does much more; it is your biggest ally in fighting sun damage, ageing, and skin cancer. Although this is a skincare guide and not a medical guide, it must be stressed: Skin cancer is a real threat. Prevention is better than cure.

All ethnic groups have more or less the same number of melanocytes – the cells that produce melanin. The difference is in how the melanocytes group and act in the body. Melanin density in the epidermis's basal layer determines skin colour.

The pigment melanin absorbs harmful UV radiation from the sun and thus protects the skin. However, too high melanin concentrations can cause hyperpigmentation, the unsightly darkening of patches of skin on the face and the body.

As often in life, one's best quality can also be your worst. Where melanin is concerned, the more melanin in your skin, the better you are protected against skin cancer. Unfortunately, the opposite is also true; the more melanin your skin has, the bigger your chances of hyperpigmentation.

It cannot be repeated enough: Staying out of the sun is the best skincare practice.

Dark Skin

Advantages

One of the most significant advantages of dark skin is that it *does not age as quickly* as other ethnic groups. Why are women with lovely ebony to dark skin so fortunate to have wrinkle-free skin until into their seventies? They have several advantages:

People with darker skin have more corneocytes in the outermost layer of the epidermis. Their cells are not significantly bigger than those of other ethnic skin types, but their corneocytes are tightly packed together. Thus, they form a solid barrier.

In addition, collagen in the dermis of people with darker skin is tightly grouped together. This firm structure adds form to the skin and contributes to looking younger.

Another advantage of darker skin is that they have *more lipids (oils) in the corneocytes.* Darker skin also has between 60 and 70% more lipids in the hair. Their sebaceous glands are also more prominent and produce more sebum (Rawlings, 2006).

Darker skin has *more melanin* than other skin colours and thus has more natural protection from UV radiation. Melanocytes produce higher amounts of melanin, which melanosomes transport to the epidermis. These melanosomes are bigger and more widely distributed in people with darker skin.

Disadvantages

There is no guarantee that people with darker skin will not burn in the sun. They might still get skin cancer and must wear sunscreen. Darker skinned people have, on average, a UVB protective factor of 13 versus that of 3 in pale-skinned people (Eucerin, 2022).

People with darker skin have *a better chance of avoiding skin cancer,* but the news is not all good. Unfortunately, many people with darker skin have a false sense of security and do not take the necessary care. They often don't go for regular skin checks. Consequently, skin cancers are picked up only in an advanced stage. This makes treatment more complex, and the outcome is not always positive.

Darker skinned people must take note: *Cancerous growths often appear on hand palms and foot soles.* As the palms and soles are usually not exposed to the sun, many people do not view these growths as dangerous.

Unfortunately, *hyperpigmentation* is very common in people with darker skin because of high melanin content. It is especially the *eye area that often turns dark*. The skin around the eyes is very thin and nearly translucent. The underlying blood vessels are thus visible and appear like dark shadows. Furthermore, the eye area is hypersensitive to pollution, an unhealthy diet, lack of sleep, and the ultimate baddies – smoking and the sun. Staring too long at your screen can also tire the eyes and worsen the shadows.

Hyperpigmentation around the eyes can also be *genetic*. If your parents had a problem with dark pigmentation around the eye, start early with creams to protect your skin. Skin lightening creams with vitamin C are effective. You will find various treatment options for hyperpigmentation in the next chapter. Some mechanical treatments, medications, and cosmetic products might worsen your problem. Be safe and instead consult a dermatologist.

One of the drawbacks of darker skin is *enlarged pore*s. This might be because of high numbers of apocrine and eccrine glands, or increased sebum secretion.

All skin types can be affected by *seborrheic dermatitis*, but the effects on darker skin are more prominent. The skin turns a light pink with greasy scales. These spots do not tan and are difficult to hide. An underlying neurological disease or immunity issue often contributes to seborrheic dermatitis. Seek professional help and do not try to treat it at home.

Skin tags, pieces of soft skin that *hang,* are bothersome and unattractive. Medical professionals have several names for them and can remove them.

Dermatosis papulosa Nigra (DPN) affects about 30% of ageing people with darker skin (Eucerin, 2022). They are small bothersome *bumps* on the face but are not dangerous. They are usually genetic, and a defect in the hair follicles is to blame. These bumps are unsightly and can be removed. However, dermatologists are generally hesitant because the wounds may cause hyperpigmentation, which might be equally unattractive.

Olive Skin

People with olive skin traditionally come from certain areas of the globe – the Middle East, the Mediterranean, South America, and Asia. About 30% of the world's population is of Asian origin (Yang, 2020). Of course, there are many skin tones in this category, and variations are the rule, not the exception. Some women have a yellower skin tone, which is the result of carotene, a chromophore.

This category includes millions of women, and each of you has to seek your own beauty. Olive-skinned women have won many of the most prestigious beauty pageants over the years. Beauties from Brazil, the Philippines, and Puerto Rico have repeatedly taken the crown away from dark and fair contestants.

Advantages

Olive-skinned people have enough *melanin* in their skin to protect them from sunburn. Some research reports suggest that on top of the presence of melanin, olive-skinned people's tolerance to UV radiation might also be attributed to diet and DNA repair enzymes.

One of the biggest advantages of olive-skinned women is the relatively high levels of the skin's own lipids – *ceramide*. Just to refresh your memory, ceramides are the skin's natural moisturisers. They are interconnected chains of carbon atoms and bind with other fatty acids to form the skin barrier. One can apply ceramides topically and thus supplement the skin's natural ceramides.

Medium-toned skin also contains more *collagen*. The dermis is thicker, another reason why medium-toned people don't show wrinkles as quickly.

Disadvantages

Olive-toned skin is prone to *sensitivity*, irritation, inflammation, and hyperpigmentation.

In general, olive-skinned women develop *hyperpigmentation* at an early age. The good news is that researchers found that women who have been using *skincare products* from a young age did not show ageing and hyperpigmentation to the same extent as those who did not use skincare products (Rawlings, 2006).

Hyperpigmentation often occurs around the *eye area, which can form dark rings*. The skin surrounding the eyes is the thinnest in your body, and the underlying blood vessels are visible. If your parents had these circles, start early in life to prevent them. Consult a dermatologist and check the next chapter for treatment options. Also, stay away from the sun and don't smoke. Get enough sleep, limit your screen time, and eat healthily. If you have a healthy lifestyle and protect yourself from the sun, you can lessen the severity of genetic hyperpigmentation.

Tape strip testing is a method researchers use to measure proteins in the skin. They apply a specialised tape multiple times on the same spot to calculate the density of components. Tape strip testing on people with olive skin proves that their skin has a weak skin barrier despite the higher ceramide content.

Research on Japanese women showed high skin sensitivity in lactic and stinging tests. Their skin also *reacted quickly*, a further indication of high sensitivity. These women had a substantial number of sweat glands, which might have contributed to their high skin sensitivity (Rawlings, 2006).

One test found that women living in the north of Japan *aged quicker* than peers living in the country's south. The women in the northern test group had a more yellow skin tone, a rougher skin texture, and less moisture in the stratum corneum (Rawlings, 2006).

Another study showed increased blood flow to a spot where researchers had applied methyl. Blood flow to the area increased, another indication of high skin sensitivity (Wan, 2014). Also, *spicy foods* and sudden *environmental changes* caused quick skin reactions (Rawlings, 2006).

Climate *and geography* impact skin quality and might have influenced some test results. Skin quality can differ from one area to another because of environmental factors. For example, people close to the equator have a higher risk of hyperpigmentation.

Fair Skin

The term 'an English rose' symbolises a typical European woman. The rose symbolises romance, and a red rose signals love. But roses don't keep long. The same goes for fair skin, which *ages fas*t. Unfortunately, like a rose, fair-skinned women might wilt soon if they do not look after their skin from early childhood.

If you have ever wondered what causes fair skin, the answer leads back to melanin. Melanin pops up all the time in this guide. In the next chapter on pigmentation, we will go even deeper into melanin. Melanin rules the roost, whether you have fair, olive, or dark skin.

Melanin – or the lack of it – is not solely responsible for the pinkish tint in fair skin. Two other chromophores, together with melanin, cause the variations of pink to red in fair-skinned people.

Advantages

But does fair skin have many physical characteristics that help protect against ageing and acne or prevent pigmentation? On the contrary, fair-skinned people *show signs of ageing earlier* than other ethnic skin types.

Fair-skinned women's risk for hyperpigmentation is slightly less because they have less melanin in their skin. They are still prone to develop melasma, hyperpigmentation, and *skin cancer* if they do not protect their skin from the sun.

Sadly, the advantages of having fair skin are often cultural, social, and economic. Even in the 21st century, people with fair skin earn higher salaries and have better health, as well as economic and educational opportunities. They are treated better at school and in the legal system.

If fair skin proves anything, it is that skincare does help. Many women with very pale skin manage to look good until their old age, despite the disadvantages of their skin type. It is proof that whatever your ethnic skin tone, *care and protection from the sun* improve skin quality.

Disadvantages

Fair-skinned people age much quicker than people with darker skin types. It boils down to melanin again. Light-skinned people have very little melanin and thus little in-built protection against UV radiation. One study reports that 55% of UVA rays penetrate lighter skin as opposed to 18% in darker skin (Hammond, 2012).

Dermatologists used a visual scoring system to assess wrinkles and found that pale-skinned women have *more wrinkles* than darker skinned women. Besides UV radiation, decreasing oestrogen levels might contribute to early ageing. Oestrogen affects the underlying structures beneath the skin and causes sagging. Sun damage causes surface wrinkling (Norton, 2010).

People with light skin often develop *age spots* on the back of their hands and face. Also called liver spots, they are benign, and you will find more information on them in the next chapter on hyperpigmentation.

Other than ageing quicker, fair-skinned people have a high risk of *skin cancer.*

In conclusion, while researching for this book, we found that every study and comment from dermatologists, cosmetic scientists, and beauty journalists stressed the importance of wearing sunscreen. The best any woman can do for her skin is to prevent UV radiation. Even if you forget everything in this book, avoid sunburn at all costs, whether you have fair, olive, or dark skin.

Quick Reminder

There is beauty in diversity: You are uniquely beautiful – not despite your skin colour but *because of your skin colour.*

It's okay to follow trends and stay fashionable, but never build your self-image on a trend.

The beauty and skincare industry does not classify skin types based on race but on their reaction to the sun.

Accept yourself and manage the challenges of your skin colour.

Don't start with make-up to improve your looks; start with skincare.

Dark-skinned women age better but are more prone to hyperpigmentation.

Olive-skinned women have more natural ceramides in their skin but are also prone to hyperpigmentation.

Fair-skinned women age quicker but are less prone to hyperpigmentation if they stay out of the sun.

Part 2: Common Skin Problems and Treatments

Let us live for the beauty of our own reality.

Chapter 5:
Pigmentation and Skin Conditions

Charles Lamb is a British author from the romantic period. He valued women and co-authored the well-known children's book *Tales from Shakespeare* with his sister, Mary Lamb. May his words 'Let us live for the beauty of our own reality' show the way for all women who have to overcome disheartening skin problems.

In Part 2 of this book, you get the opportunity to face your skin challenges and accept them as your reality. The following chapters will help you identify not only your skin problem but the exact nature of this problem. It will also help you determine the cause and give you treatment options.

Work With Your Own Reality

So what is your skin's reality? If you are reading this book, chances are you or a loved one is probably faced with the reality of a skin problem, a condition that spoils one's looks, ruins one's social life, and crushes self-esteem. The first step in overcoming the issue is to get help. Do not hide away from the world. Yes, it is difficult to see other women with flawless skin having fun while your skin seems to put people off.

If you are embarrassed and feel isolated because of your skin, seek help immediately. You are probably already spending money on over-the-counter medications that do not help. The sooner you get professional help on board, the sooner your physical and emotional healing can start. There is no quick cure, and the longer you delay, the longer you will hide from the world.

Take courage from the fact that your skin is dynamic and new cells always form. In younger women, it takes about a month to move from the dermis through all the sub-layers to the stratum corneum, where they are shed. In older women, the process takes longer, but your skin is alive. Its regenerative ability proves it will improve with the proper treatment. Remember, though, that your skin cells must undergo several renewing cycles before it heals completely.

The next step is getting an accurate diagnosis of your skin problem. It's not enough to know you have unsightly brown patches on your face. To treat it correctly, you must know what caused the discolouring in the first place. The same goes for acne, unwanted facial hair, or signs of premature ageing. You can only get the proper treatment when you know what caused the problem in the first place.

Get Professional Help

Sometimes the pigmentation seems to come from nowhere, and you might wonder where you went wrong. If your pigmentation is bad enough to affect your self-esteem, seek the help of a dermatologist, preferably someone who specialises in the field of hyperpigmentation. Dermatologists train for many years and are best equipped to identify the cause of your pigmentation and can treat the specific type of pigmentation. They can also advise on how to prevent further damage.

Earlier chapters discussed the Fitzpatrick and Baumann systems for classifying skin type. The Roberts hyperpigmentation scale is a seven-point system specialising in hyperpigmentation. Dermatologists use the Roberts scale to determine what type of hyperpigmentation you struggle with. Although the treatments are similar, each type has its own challenges. The doctor will also examine your skin and ask about your medical history and ancestral background. This information will determine the best treatment and ways to prevent further damage.

Hyperpigmentation may cause scarring. The Roberts scarring scale determines the possibility of long-term scarring caused by pigmentation. Certain medicines and cosmetic procedures, such as chemical peels, Intense Pulsed Light (IPL), and hair removal might contribute to scarring. If you're prone to scarring, the doctor will adjust your treatment and advise you on safe mechanical treatment.

Pigmentation, Hyperpigmentation, and Hypopigmentation

You might be confused by the different terms used in skincare.

- Pigmentation is the skin's natural colouring, usually after an injury or blisters. This type of pigmentation is typically temporary and will disappear over time.

- Hyperpigmentation is a collective term and includes several skin conditions that cause dark patches on the skin. It is not dangerous but can be unattractive and often emotionally devastating.

- Hypopigmentation happens when there is not enough melanin in the skin, resulting in flat white patches.

Hyperpigmentation and the Sun

Not all skin types react to sun exposure in the same way. The skin's reaction to UV radiation is so important that Fitzpatrick used it as the basis for his skin classification system more than 50 years ago. This system is still in use, which proves how important it is to avoid sun damage. Furthermore, the skin's reaction to the sun indicates its susceptibility to pigmentation, irritations, and inflammation.

Melanin is both an ally and a baddie when it comes to skin quality, but melanin is only dangerous when the skin suffers sunburn. The desire to tan and our love of the outdoors can harm our skin.

The terms SPF, UV radiation, UVA, UVB, and UVC are confusing. The first refers to the level of protection, and the last three are harmful radiation types. Hopefully, knowledge about the damage they can do to your skin will motivate you to wear sunscreen, big hats, and sunglasses.

- SPF stands for Sun Protection Factor and measures how much UV radiation (sunlight) will be needed to burn skin *that is already protected by sunscreen.*

- UV radiation is the sun's rays. It has three grades of rays: UVA, UVB, and UVC.

- UVA has the lowest energy but higher wavelengths. They penetrate deeper and affect the cells in the epidermis and dermis. They even cause damage to your DNA. They cause wrinkles, ageing, and potentially skin cancer. The ozone does not absorb UVA rays; consequently, UVA rays cause about 95% of sunburn. They can even burn you through windows and clouds. Tanning beds use predominantly UVAs.

- UVB has a medium energy level and shorter wavelengths. Although they only burn the cells in the top layer of the skin, they damage your DNA and cause most skin cancers. The ozone absorbs UVBs only partially. Tanning beds use UVB in combination with UVA. Fortunately, UVB rays do not penetrate windows or clouds.

- UVC has the highest energy level and the shortest wavelengths. They affect only the outer layer of the epidermis. Thankfully, clouds filter most UVC rays before they reach the ground.

Types of Hyperpigmentation

Melasma

Melasma is the most common type of pigmentation, often called the 'mask of pregnancy'. However, not only pregnant women have melasma. It has several causes: UV radiation, hormones, or the side effects of certain drugs. Superficial melasma might disappear within months if you diligently wear sunscreen and stay out of the sun as much as possible.

Persistent or severe melasma requires medical attention. The dermatologist will use a specialised light to see whether the damaged cells have penetrated your dermis. He might even do a small skin biopsy, a quick and harmless procedure.

Furthermore, it is essential to identify the triggers that cause your melasma: birth control pills, prolonged stress, or over-exposure to sunlight. For example, sportswomen who spend long hours on the sports field should reapply sunscreen every two hours.

Post-Inflammatory Hyperpigmentation (PIH)

The psychological effects of post-inflammatory hyperpigmentation are devastating. This pigmentation can occur after an injury, prolonged acne, or skin inflammation. The result is heavily discoloured patches on previously infected areas.

The skin automatically increases melanin production to help heal inflammation. When the skin gets inflamed, melanin is produced to fight the inflammation. It is thus a defence mechanism to protect the skin. Unfortunately, the worse your inflammation is, the higher melanin secretion becomes and the worse your pigmentation might be.

Unfortunately, many acne sufferers develop hyperpigmentation, adding additional emotional stress. Many people feel they are doubly punished – first acne and then hyperpigmentation. It is immensely discouraging, but don't despair. It seems unfair, but you have succeeded in winning the fight against acne. If you have won over acne, you can win this fight also. Your pigmentation will not disappear overnight, but you don't have to go through life feeling stigmatised.

Hyperpigmentation targets both genders, and people with dark skin (Fitzpatrick types 3 to 6) are more at risk because they have more natural melanin.

Let's look at a simplified version of how melanin is formed in the skin:

- The melanocytes produce skin pigments (melanin, eumelanin, and pheomelanin). To prevent confusion, we use the term melanin only.

- Melanosomes in the melanocyte carry the melanin pigment to the keratinocytes.

- The keratinocytes move upward to the stratum corneum. Each melanin-producing cell – melanocyte – is attached to at least 30 keratinocytes.

- The stratum corneum is what others see, and it consists mostly of keratinocytes. They form dark patches when inflamed.

It cannot be stressed enough: Stay out of the sun. UV radiation will worsen your condition.

Hyperpigmentation will eventually fade, but the process is very slow. Without treatment, it can take many years, depending on the severity of the discolouration. Fortunately, it does not cause scarring, and a good foundation could hide the worst. Make-up is seldom a solution to a skin problem, but in this case, get the best coverage you can afford. Use a concealer that does not block your pores. Consult a beautician who does not sell a specific brand for the best concealer to suit your skin colour.

Treatment of Post-Inflammatory Hyperpigmentation

Treatment options for hyperpigmentation follow later in this chapter. Not all treatments are suitable for all types of hyperpigmentation. Your doctor will recommend a treatment based on your specific problem, the kind of discolouring, your health, and your genetic background.

Do not rush into any treatment because it has worked for somebody else. Some topical and mechanical treatments can trigger an overproduction of melanin. Instead of improving your skin, you might worsen your condition.

Age Spots

Age spots are also called liver spots. The medical name is 'solar lentiginosis'. They often appear on the backs of the hands and faces of older light-skinned people, especially those with blue eyes. The spots are flat and oval-shaped. They vary between brown, grey, and black.

They are harmless but unsightly. Treat age spots the same as other types of hyperpigmentation. A lightening cream might also contain retinol and cosmetic bleach. Do not try household bleach at home; it can scar you.

Hyperpigmentation Treatment Options

Sunscreen

Protection from the sun is your first-line treatment against all types of pigmentation. Even if you will be outdoors for a short period, wear a wide-brimmed hat and refresh your sunscreen regularly. Good sunscreens contain zinc oxide, titanium dioxide, and iron dioxide. Don't be alarmed by the names; an oxide is a binary compound of oxygen and another element – not harmful at all.

Anti-Inflammatory Diet

Your shopping basket might be the key to persistent inflammation that contributes to hyperpigmentation. And for coffee lovers, a limited number of coffees is good for fighting inflammation. Coffee has anti-inflammatory compounds, information you might find handy if anybody dares to criticise your coffee habit in the future.

Inflammation is a natural process in the body meant to fight foreign invaders. As soon as your body picks up a threat, your immune system starts inflammation to attack the harmful substance. When the immune system does not stop the inflammation once the danger has passed, it becomes chronic inflammation.

Substances in natural foods – predominantly plants and fruits – can stop chronic inflammation.

Unfortunately, some foods – white bread, pastries, chips, sugary drinks, red meat, processed foods, and margarine – feed inflammation.

Many doctors recommend a Mediterranean diet high in fruit, vegetables, whole grains, fish, nuts, and olive oil. The Mediterranean diet contributes to weight control and emotional well-being.

Lightening Creams

Lightening creams are skin bleachers and can be dangerous. Health authorities have regulated them during the past decades because of severe health risks. They might cause kidney and neurological damage and are only available on prescription. Examples are hydroquinone, mercury, and high doses of steroids. Over-the-counter creams might even worsen your pigmentation. Also, be careful when using two or more products together, as they can cause adverse side effects.

It cannot be stressed enough: Refrain from self-treatment. Your dermatologist's advice is an investment in your skin health, and the doctor might prescribe a safe lightening cream for hyperpigmentation.

- Hydroquinone, a powerful topical treatment, is so potent that over-the-counter products may not contain it. A dermatologist will evaluate your skin and general health before prescribing hydroquinone.

- Tretinoin is a well-known acne treatment and is prescribed for pigmentation marks also. It is a concentrated form of retinol and keeps the pores open and clean. It is often combined with a low corticosteroid dose. Corticosteroid is an anti-inflammatory that will lighten the dark pigmentation over time.

- In severe cases, the dermatologist might prescribe a cream that contains hydroquinone, tretinoin, and corticosteroid. It is called triple combination and is highly effective – on the condition that you never leave the house without sunscreen.

- In severe cases, tranexamic acid might be prescribed. It is relatively new in hyperpigmentation treatment, but doctors have prescribed it for heavy menstrual bleeding for many years. In topical form, it alters the way cells produce melanin. You might see a reduction in dark spots within three months. It also does not have many side effects. A 2022 study reported positive results specifically for post-inflammatory hyperpigmentation (Strong, 2022).

- Patients often take tranexamic acid with the triple combination cream mentioned above for even better results.

- If your pigmentation is not severe, a gentle medication such as vitamin C, azelaic acid, liquorice acid, arbutin or kojic acid will help. Kojic acid is naturally found in mild form in some mushrooms and fermented rice. Arbutin comes from the bearberry plant and stops the growth of melanin production. Be safe, and consult a dermatologist before you use any of these.

Mechanical Treatment

Mechanical treatments help and are usually repeated over several sessions.

It can be costly, though, and is best done by a dermatologist or a trained professional. Check whether the beautician is fully trained and has professional registration. An unqualified person might not have the scientific background and could harm your skin, even cause scarring.

Also, these treatments are effective only if you stay out of the sun. Mechanical treatments take off the outermost layer of the stratum corneum. *Exposure to the sun will cause even more damage, and the discoloured patches will worsen.* If you decide on any of the following treatments, you have to commit to using sunscreen when outside.

- A chemical peel is uncomfortable but effective when repeated over months. The acid dissolves the topmost skin on the stratum corneum. It stimulates the new cells to move upward, and the damaged cells are shed. A series of treatments are necessary, but staying out of the sun during treatment is vital, and you must avoid exposure for the rest of your life.

- Microneedling is a minimum-invasive procedure that causes extremely fine wounds on the skin surface. The doctor uses ultrathin needles during this process; consequently, the wounds are microscopic. Still, they signal the skin to produce collagen. New cells move upward to heal the tiny incisions, and your skin is rejuvenated.

- Laser and light treatments heat and destroy melanin in the skin. The spots will initially become darker before they flake and shed. There are different types of laser treatments, and the doctor will recommend the type most suitable for your specific pigmentation problem. Laser technology is highly specialised and expensive. If you go this route, trust your dermatologist and give your full cooperation by taking precautions when you go outside.

  o Also known as fractionated laser treatment, it causes minute injuries to the skin's outermost layer. The pigment is destroyed, but the skin reacts by producing more collagen, which heals the affected area. You will need several treatments and also to go for regular maintenance sessions.

o Underlying blood vessels contribute to stubborn hyperpigmentation, and fractionated laser resurfacing helps deliver targeted drugs to the area. This new development brings hope to people who have tried many treatments without satisfying results. If you suffer from persistent hyperpigmentation, this might be the next step.

o A broad-band light laser uses heat waves of varying lengths. It is used for patients with brown pigmentation spots and background redness because of dilated capillaries.

• The injection of platelet-rich plasma offers a different treatment option. The dermatologist takes a small blood sample and separates the plasma from other substances in the blood in a centrifuge machine. The plasma is rich in growth factors and is injected into the skin. These growth factors stimulate collagen production, which helps to even out the discolouring. It is a new method but shows positive results in treating hyperpigmentation.

Hypopigmentation

Hypopigmentation – light, flat patches on the skin – happens when the melanocytes do not produce melanin. There are different types of hypopigmentation.

Skin Injuries

Wounds, blisters, infection, and burning often result in a lighter patch on the skin. The trauma damages the melanocytes, and they temporarily do not produce melanin. Natural melanin production will occur once the skin's inner layers have healed. Immediately after injury, The surface wound might look healed, as white blood cells immediately move in and seal the wound to keep harmful bacteria out. However, the inner layers of the skin take a bit longer to heal.

Be patient and cover the light area with make-up specially designed for the purpose. There are several products on the market, but make sure you use one that does not contain any harmful ingredients.

Vitiligo: Autoimmune Disorder

Vitiligo is an autoimmune disorder that damages pigment-producing melanocytes. People with darker skin are more prone to develop vitiligo, and children of parents with vitiligo have a larger chance of developing it.

Unfortunately, there is no cure for it. Still, researchers are investigating new topical treatments: Janus kinase inhibitor is a drug that regulates enzyme activity in the skin, which might be helpful for vitiligo and several other skin diseases.

It often starts when injuries are exposed to the sun or harmful chemicals. The Vitiligo Research Foundation, a member of the United Nations Economica and Social Council, operates globally. The Foundation reports that vitiligo affects 1 out of every 100 people and can cause severe emotional trauma and social isolation.

Treatment

The sooner treatment starts, the better the chances of healing are. Treatment varies from camouflaging the patches with special make-up, restoring the pigmentation, or letting the skin go completely white.

Repigmentation is a long process; the later treatment starts, the harder it is to reverse. Parents should seek help immediately if a child shows prominent flat white patches. The dermatologist will assess the patient's family history, age, type of vitiligo, where it is located on the body, and general health.

Light therapy is effective, but the process is long, and it can take up to two years to restore pigmentation to the area. Self-diagnosis and self-treatment can be dangerous; see a professional for help.

Albinism

Albinism is an inherited disease with an abnormal gene affecting the melanin enzyme. The skin, hair, and eyes have no colour, and sun exposure is the biggest risk.

People with albinism often have vision problems, which can be corrected or improved by assistance from an optician.

There is no treatment to cure albinism. Protection from UV radiation is vital to prevent skin damage and cancer:

- sunglasses to protect the eyes from UV rays
- protective clothing
- sunscreen

Skin Conditions Your Doctor Can Help With

Mariska Hargitay, the strong female detective in *Law and Order*, said in a somewhat different context: 'Healing takes time, and asking for help is a courageous step'.

Her words also apply to people with skin conditions. A flawed skin can make life unbearable, but you don't have to suffer and live with the problem. A dermatologist can help.

Environmental factors such as allergens, fungi, medication, viruses, bacteria, and the sun cause many skin conditions. Fortunately, modern dermatology uses advanced diagnostic methods to accurately determine the type of disease and its cause. These diagnostic methods include biopsies, skin patch tests, microscope slides, a hand-held dermoscopy, and a Tzanck test designed to test for herpes viruses.

People with diabetes, inflammatory bowel disease, lupus, or who are on certain medications are prone to skin conditions. They should inform the dermatologist of their health issues, including chronic medicines. Some chronic conditions might improve with treatment but return after remission. In such cases, treatment will have to be repeated from time to time, but you will at least know what it is and what to expect.

- Actinic keratosis is a scaly skin patch caused by long-term sun exposure. It is a pre-cancer warning to be taken seriously.

- Athlete's foot is a fungus infection and causes itching, redness, and cracked skin. The toenails change colour, becoming white, yellow, or brown, and disintegrate.

- Alopecia areata is an autoimmune condition that causes patchy hair loss on the scalp, body, and chin.

- Atopic dermatitis (eczema) results in dry, itchy skin that cracks and is primarily seen in children. The good news is that children usually outgrow eczema.

- Basal cell carcinoma presents as red, scaly spots on areas usually exposed to the sun. They are curable; see your doctor as soon as possible. Depending on the severity, the dermatologist will treat it either topically or remove it surgically.

- A viral infection causes cold sores; blisters that develop around the mouth. It starts with a tingling sensation, then becomes red and filled with fluid. It can take up to three weeks to heal. You might also experience fever, headaches, and a sore throat. The herpes simplex virus might be dormant in nerve cells and emerge when you have a fever, suffer from prolonged stress, or are overtired.

- Hives are itchy swellings caused by insect bites, food, or medication. They usually disappear after a few hours, but chronic urticaria can be very uncomfortable. If you know what caused your hives, it can be avoided.

- Psoriasis is caused by a compromised immune system and can be triggered by cold weather, stress, infections, injuries, beta-blocker drugs, alcohol, and smoking. People with darker skin develop purple patches with grey scaling, while people with lighter skin have pinkish patches with silvery scaling.

- Rosacea, a chronic red swelling accompanied by pimples, is the bane of many women. It is caused by an immune system that does not function 100 percent and is aggravated by environmental irritations.

- Shingles in adults can be painful and cause significant discomfort, especially in older adults or those with other chronic diseases. The chickenpox virus, herpes zoster, causes shingles accompanied by fever, fatigue, and headaches.

- Warts are skin growths caused by viruses that are spread by direct person-t0-person contact. Salicylic acid is an over-the-counter treatment available as a gel or a pad.

Quick Reminder

Hyperpigmentation can destroy your self-image and life. Don't hide but seek professional advice.

The primary causes are over-exposure to the sun, hormonal imbalances, and inflammation. These factors cause an overproduction of melanin, which results in unsightly discolouring.

If your hyperpigmentation is severe and persistent, consult a dermatologist.

There are different types of hyperpigmentation, and each type has different causes. Therefore, treatment is adapted accordingly.

The types of hyperpigmentation are: melasma, post-inflammatory hyperpigmentation, and age spots.

Treatment options include: consistently wearing sunscreen in summer and winter, following an anti-inflammatory diet, skin lighteners (applied topically and prescribed by a dermatologist), mechanical treatments (done by a dermatologist and, in some cases, beauticians), and platelet-rich plasma injections (only done by a doctor).

Hypopigmentation caused by injuries to the skin will eventually heal.

The sooner vitiligo is treated, the better the chances are of preventing it from spreading.

There are medical treatments for most skin conditions. They need not cause you embarrassment or spoil your appearance and social life.

Chapter 6:
Acne – Not a Life Sentence

The absence of flaw in beauty is itself a flaw.

Havelock Ellis was a medical doctor who studied human sexuality. Far ahead of his time, he co-authored a medical textbook on homosexuality in 1897. Ellis's words are an encouragement to any woman who suffers from acne.

Acne is not a life sentence. You can overcome acne, and *knowledge* is the best weapon to address this 'flaw'. It is important to determine the cause of your acne, as not all types of acne are treated the same. It is important not to treat acne on the skin surface only but to address the underlying problem that causes your acne. Fight your acne with facts. There is life after acne!

Those lucky ones who never had more than a few pimples in their teens won't understand acne's devastating effects. The rest of us know: Acne causes intense emotional trauma, deep-seated insecurity, and a feeling of worthlessness. Dermatologists worldwide report that acne is the biggest single skin problem for patients of all ages.

If you suffer from acne, a dermatologist will help heal the physical lesions on your face, even though it could take months. But many acne sufferers have deep emotional scars also. Your dermatologist will lead you to healthy skin, but he is not trained to heal your inner scars. Nonetheless, dermatologists are acutely aware of how acne affects their patients. Even if the patient appears calm, their body language reveals the truth. Some avoid eye contact, others hide their anxiety behind jokes or aloofness. In many cases, your dermatologist might advise you to see a counsellor.

Once you have taken the step to seek medical help, speak to a psychologist or counsellor who can help you recover emotionally also. A psychologist might use the Quality of Life (QoL) scale to test your emotional well-being. These scales are designed to test for factors that impact your quality of life; they do not analyse your character or delve deep into your psyche. They are designed to help, not to upset you further.

Don't hesitate to get help, especially if you experience any of the following: loss of appetite, lethargy, mood disturbances, sleep disturbances, feeling unworthy, spontaneous crying, depression, or suicidal thoughts.

Psychological Effects on Adolescents

Acne affects 30 to 50% of adolescents (Fried, 2013).

Poets often compare youth to spring, blossoms, new life, and love. Young people with acne experience the exact opposite. This crucial stage of their lives is often a nightmare, and they feel like their lives have ended before they have even reached adulthood. The burden of acne is the last thing a teenager needs.

Adolescence is a difficult time for young people. Their bodies change, and their emotions fluctuate continuously. They become more independent from their parents and seek peer acceptance. Unfortunately, the opposite sometimes happens, and kids with acne are often bullied at school and suffer intense humiliation.

Adolescence is a psychologically vulnerable phase, and bullying because of acne causes intense feelings of isolation, anxiety, and depression. These kids avoid social gatherings and sports activities. Instead of forming closer relationships with friends, poor body image hinders their social development.

Quite often, their schoolwork deteriorates. They miss assignments and stay away from school to escape the humiliation of being called out because of their appearance.

The unemployment rate is also higher in young people with moderate to severe acne. They might perform poorly in job interviews because of low self-esteem; employers are often biassed and pass over applicants with severe acne.

Acne destroys the quality of life of thousands of young people. But there are treatments available that can improve acne. This chapter will help you determine the cause of your acne and also give an overview of available treatments.

Psychological Effects on Adults

Not only young people suffer under the burden of acne. Adult acne is common and equally as devastating to self-image and self-confidence. Adults also experience high levels of emotional distress and social anxiety. Many women avoid social events, which contributes to loneliness and unhappiness. Understandably, they sometimes feel robbed of normal, happy relationships and are angry at life.

But how prevalent is adult acne among women?

German dermatologists report increased female adult acne since the turn of the century (Dreno, 2018). Acne is a sword hanging over acne sufferers' private and professional lives.

Especially females' self-esteem is linked to their appearance, and acne causes self-consciousness and social isolation. Very often, it also impacts personal relationships, as the sufferer feels unattractive and does not believe herself worthy of love.

The work environment is seldom sympathetic, and adult sufferers regularly report difficulty gaining employment. Those in jobs often feel stigmatised and isolated and struggle to get promotions.

It is no wonder that many women are deeply depressed and have suicidal thoughts. If you are in this category, take your first step toward recovery and a full life by getting at the cause of your acne. Knowledge is power, and knowing the reason for your acne is the first step in getting the proper treatment.

What Is Acne?

Acne has no respect for age, gender, or ethnic group. It affects 9,4% of the global population and rates eighth among the world's most prevalent diseases (Tan, 2015). Another source reports that 50 million Americans have acne (Cleveland Clinic, 2022).

In contrast to many other diseases, acne does not impair one's functionality. The individual suffers, but life goes on for everybody else. Acne sufferers feel as if their world has become unbearable.

Acne usually starts in puberty but can continue well into adulthood. But where does it all start?

It starts in the sebaceous glands in the skin. Both genders have increased levels of the male sex hormones (androgens) in puberty. Androgens stimulate the sebaceous glands, and they secrete more sebum.

The sebaceous glands and sebum play a vital role as a natural moisturiser in the skin. The sebum moves up in the hair follicle and exits through the pore. Sebum is the body's in-built moisturiser and the natural way to keep the skin hydrated.

The trouble starts when dead cells and other substances block the pores. Natural bacteria feed on the sebum in the hair follicle. The body's immune system gets ready to fight when the bacteria in a plugged follicle multiply out of control. The immune system regards any bacteria concentration as a danger. It sends white blood cells to the hair follicle to secrete an enzyme to kill the bacteria. Unfortunately, these enzymes can also damage the wall of the hair follicle.

The result is acne: the dreaded skin condition that spoils your appearance and destroys your self-esteem.

There are several types of acne, and these are grouped into *comedo acne* and *inflammatory lesions*. Comedones are open or closed pores and, though bothersome, are seldom severe. Inflammatory acne is often painful and can cause scarring and hyperpigmentation.

TYPES OF ACNE

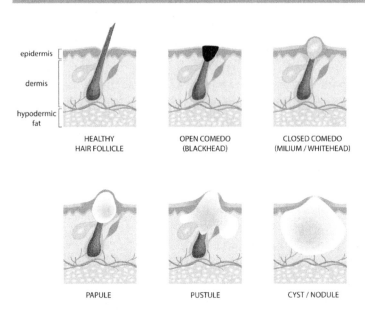

epidermis

dermis

hypodermic fat

HEALTHY
HAIR FOLLICLE

OPEN COMEDO
(BLACKHEAD)

CLOSED COMEDO
(MILIUM / WHITEHEAD)

PAPULE

PUSTULE

CYST / NODULE

Comedones

Blackheads

Blackheads appear on the nose and chin, the oily areas of the skin. So-called male hormones (androgens) stimulate the sebaceous glands to secrete more sebum. Too much sebum blocks the pores, and bacteria get active in the hair follicle. Keratin, the protein found in hair and nails, also becomes overactive, contributing to even more blackhead formation.

Blackheads are not inflammatory acne, as they do not have pus. Blackheads are small bumps with openings at the surface.

Because they are black, many people think they are dirty, but it is untrue. They look black on the skin surface because the sebum turns dark when it is exposed to air.

Blackheads, just like all other types of acne, can affect your physical appearance and self-confidence. Do not suffer unnecessarily; you can treat blackheads successfully with non-prescription topical applications: salicylic acid, azelaic acid, benzoyl peroxide, and various retinoid forms. You will find more information on these topical applications below.

Although unattractive, most blackheads heal more readily than other types of acne as they are close to the surface.

When your blackheads are deeply buried in your skin, you need professional help, as they might not go away on their own. Therefore, see a dermatologist if your blackheads are persistent and do not improve with over-the-counter products. Your emotional wellness is at stake, and the doctor can prescribe antibiotics and more potent retinoids.

Also, consider salon treatments such as chemical peels and laser skin resurfacing.

Whiteheads

Whiteheads are also comedo acne. They are unattractive and annoying but can be treated and prevented. They form when dead cells, oil, and bacteria settle in a closed pore. Whiteheads differ from blackheads in that they are closed under a thin cover that looks white.

Pores become clogged because of too high sebum levels, especially when the body undergoes hormonal changes. It happens typically during puberty, menstruation, pregnancy, or even as a side effect of birth control medications. Unfortunately, your genes sometimes also play a role in the overproduction of sebum.

Whiteheads are a milder form of acne and can also be treated with topical retinoids. Don't expect immediate improvement, though. Retinoids remove the outermost dead cells, and this process can take up to three months. Sunscreen is vital if you use any cream or lotion with retinoids, as your skin will be more sensitive to sun damage.

Doctors might also prescribe an oral contraceptive to reduce whiteheads, especially if you also have other types of acne.

Inflammatory Acne

Inflammatory acne is red and painful. The term inflammatory acne includes papules, pustules, nodular, and cystic acne. They are caused by inflammation but are different in appearance and are treated differently. In moderate to severe cases, you must see a dermatologist.

Papules

Papules are solid, conical bumps, usually smaller than one centimetre. Some are skin-coloured but they can also be red, brown, or purple. They are easily recognisable, commonly appear during adolescence, and might continue into adulthood.

Although papules are caused by inflammation, they are not pus-filled. As with other forms of acne, papules are caused by excess sebum secretion. Hormonal imbalances, increased bacteria, and medications such as corticosteroids and anabolic steroids also contribute to papules. Your genes might also play a role in your papules.

Mild papule flare-ups usually disappear within days. Resist squeezing a pimple. You will only prolong the outbreak and will do more harm than good. External bacteria can enter the papule and worsen the inflammation. You might even end up with scarring and hyperpigmentation.

You can get over-the-counter treatments such as azelaic acid, benzoyl peroxide, retinoids, and salicylic acid. If you have persistent and painful papules, your doctor can prescribe oral and topical antibiotics. Another option is anti-androgens, which are only available on prescription.

Pustules

Pustules and papules differ in that pustules, as their name indicates, have pus. Papules are inflamed but do not ooze pus. However, papules can develop into pustules.

A pustule is a big pimple and a sign of underlying inflammation. As with all acne types, pustules are caused by overactive sebaceous glands and excess sebum production. Hormonal imbalances during puberty are often to blame. Pustules may develop into cysts and become painful. See your doctor when this happens; cystic acne can cause scarring.

Skin infections like smallpox can also cause pustules. The sudden onset of many pustules usually indicates an underlying infection that needs medical attention.

Over-the-counter treatments are usually effective in milder cases. Try benzoyl peroxide, salicylic acid, and sulphur. A bacterial infection probably causes pustules if your condition does not improve with over-the-counter treatments. In this case, get medical help. The doctor will prescribe oral and/or topical antibiotics for pustules caused by bacterial infections.

In severe cases, photodynamic therapy (PDT) might help. You will find more information on photodynamic therapy below.

Nodular Acne

These are lumps just under the skin or even deeper in the skin tissue. They are painful with a red surface but do not have a yellow or black centre. Nodules are caused by inflammation, and you cannot self-treat them. They can cause severe scarring.

The dermatologist will advise you on the best treatment option and might prescribe a combination of isotretinoin (orally taken) and benzoyl peroxide (topically applied).

Doctors sometimes treat large, persistent nodules with cortisone injections. These injections are done when nodules do not react to other treatments. The doctor uses a fine needle and injects cortisone directly into the nodule. Unfortunately, cortisone has adverse side effects, and an injection is usually a last resort. However, cortisone injections are effective and clear inflammation quickly, which speeds up the healing.

Nodules are firm and painful. Like other pimples, it is caused by the bacterium Cutibacterium acnes (C acnes), which is trapped under the skin and causes inflammation. Nodules can also have several other causes: excessive sweating, hormones, oily skin and hair products, stress, and anxiety. Medication that includes corticosteroids might also cause nodular acne.

Unfortunately, nodules can also be genetic, but you can still treat them.

Cystic Acne

Nodular and cystic acne are painful lumps that form under the skin but differ considerably. Cysts are somewhat softer and filled with fluid. You will know the difference because cysts usually ooze pus, while nodules are firmer with no fluid. Acne sufferers often have both.

The treatment for cysts and nodules overlap, but your doctor might prescribe oral and topical antibiotics for cysts, as they can scar your skin. Adapalene, tretinoin, and tazarotene are retinoids that help remove the dead cells from the skin's outermost layer. Retinoids open the pores and lessen inflammation.

When cysts are persistent, your doctor might also inject corticosteroid or, in extreme cases, prescribe isotretinoin. Isotretinoin can be dangerous. Please read the information later in this chapter carefully.

Squeezing a yellow pus-filled pimple seems tempting. Do not squeeze. Cysts often cause cellulitis, a bacterial infection that causes scarring and hyperpigmentation. These scars and dark spots might stay on your face for up to a year. Thus, don't squeeze; be patient and follow the doctor's advice to a T.

Acne Causes

The causes of acne are predominantly the same in puberty and adulthood: excess sebum, clogged pores, bacteria, and underlying inflammation.

Hormones

Hormonal changes mark the human lifecycle. It starts in the womb and carries on well into adulthood. Medical practitioners don't use the term 'hormonal acne'. Still, in layperson's terms, hormonal acne refers to hormonal changes in the body from childhood to old age: puberty, menstruation, pregnancy, and menopause.

The reproductive system starts developing during puberty, and sex hormones, among them androgens, are released. Although androgens are seen as male hormones, all genders have androgens. The best-known androgen is testosterone.

Let's recap quickly: An increase in androgens triggers sebum production. Bacteria flourishes in the excess sebum in the hair follicle. The follicle opening, the pore, becomes blocked, and the immune system reacts to irritants through inflammation. However, inflammation does not always stop in time and can damage the cell membrane: The result is acne.

Women can get acne even during menopause because of hormonal changes. Menopausal women with acne usually have normal testosterone levels but less oestrogen, which contributes to acne. Sadly, many grandmothers suffer from acne along with their granddaughters.

Stress

Stress can have devastating consequences for women with acne. Stress wears a catch-22 hat when it comes to acne. Stress releases hormones that could contribute to acne; negative emotions because of acne cause stress. It is a vicious circle: Acne causes stress, and stress activates the secretion of hormones that directly or indirectly contribute to acne. And acne causes more stress!

When excess stress hormones such as adrenaline and cortisol are secreted, they block the pores. Furthermore, stress leads to disturbed sleep patterns, immunity disorders, and menstrual cycle disturbances – adding to stress levels.

Unfortunately, stress also leads to comfort eating. If a woman feels unattractive, she often overeats. She inadvertently gains weight, which causes insulin and leptin levels to go haywire. They contribute to inflammation, which worsens acne.

If you are unsure about the cause of your acne, take note of your flair-ups. Do they coincide with periods of intense stress? For example, is your acne worse in times of intense emotional or professional stress? Some women often get off a long flight with unexplained bumps on their faces.

Prolonged emotional stress can cause acne. If you suspect stress causes your acne, see a therapist. Medical assistance alone will not help if you neglect to address the core problem.

Environmental Factors

Environmental factors, such as high humidity, can contribute to acne. The skin is abnormally hot and sweaty in humid conditions. The sweat does not evaporate rapidly because the air is too humid. The sebaceous glands work harder, and the pores clog more rapidly.

In an article published by *Frontiers in Public Health* in 2020, the authors report a 5,1% increase in global acne, attributed to worsening air pollution, a diet high in sugars, an unhealthy lifestyle, and population densities in cities (Yang, 2020).

Cosmetic and skincare products containing high percentages of lanolin, petroleum, and vegetable oils might be too oily for acne-prone skin. Check the ingredients on your products and switch to oil-free products.

In rare cases, exposure to fungicides, herbicides, insecticides, and wood preservatives can worsen acne.

Diet

Although scientists suspect diet might affect acne, not enough research has been done to prove it. Yet, foods high in glycaemic acid seem to worsen acne.

Here is a simplified explanation of the theory: The glycaemic index measures how carbohydrates affect blood sugar levels. Carbohydrates such as white bread, pastries, white rice, pasta, sugar, and sweeteners release sugar in the blood. The body secretes insulin to change sugar into energy. Foods high in carbohydrates (high-glycaemic foods) release high amounts of sugar, and the body secretes more insulin to convert the excess sugar into energy.

However, insulin activates androgen hormones and the insulin growth factor (IGF) that also boosts sebum production.

To illustrate just how complicated the link between diet and acne is, let us look at the influence your cappuccino might have on your acne.

If you love a frothy cappuccino, you will be glad to hear that cow milk has a low glycaemic index. That is good, isn't it? A low glycaemic index means milk is not bad for acne.

Don't order a second cup yet; milk contributes to acne in many ways.

- Milk contains androgens. Androgens affect sebum production and speed up the process during which keratinocytes move to the skin surface, become hard, dry, and eventually die. Increased keratinisation might clog pores even more.

- The amino acids in milk produce insulin when you take them with carbohydrates. And insulin activates the production of yet more androgen.

- Whey proteins and iodine in milk contribute to blackheads and whiteheads.

Experts are unanimous in their verdict that diets high in fats are bad. Fats contribute to weight gain, high blood pressure, and many other killer diseases. Dieticians suspect fast foods also worsen acne.

Just to add to the complexity of research regarding the link between diet and acne:

- The sebaceous glands need fatty acids to form sebum. Monounsaturated fatty acids in vegetable oils are healthy and reduce cholesterol levels, but they increase sebum production.

- Other fatty acids, again, unblock follicles and reduce sebum production.

- Foods rich in Omega-6 fats such as soy oils probably contribute to acne.

Scientists agree more research is needed to understand the role diet plays in acne. Nonetheless, a low-glycaemic diet with limited proteins, fat, and dairy benefits acne sufferers.

Until more scientific evidence comes to the fore, eat moderate amounts of dairy, meat, and proteins, but avoid sugars. Iodine and zinc seem to help with pustules; thus, make sure you add the following to your diet: low-fat milk, yoghurt, chickpeas, kidney beans, and baked beans. Some manufacturers add zinc to cereals and oats. Check the labels before buying.

And now for the million-dollar question: What about chocolate? Is there a link between chocolate and acne? Several informal studies have positively linked chocolate to increased acne, but there is no conclusion yet. In the meantime, employ moderation in all things – unfortunately, also when having chocolate.

Side Effects From Medications

Most acne cases are not related to medications, but there are exceptions. If you are on any of the following, *speak to your doctor and/or dermatologist* to ensure that you have interpreted the label correctly: corticosteroids, lithium, anticonvulsants, barbiturates, androgenic steroids, and DHEA.

- Corticosteroids are prescribed for asthma, hay fever, hives, atopic eczema, chronic obstructive pulmonary disease, inflamed joints, muscles, and tendons, lupus, inflammatory bowel disease, Crohn's disease, and ulcerative colitis.

- Lithium is often used to treat mania and bipolar disorder.

- Anticonvulsants are used to treat epilepsy, brain disorders, and migraine prevention.

- Barbiturates are used for anxiety, insomnia, and some seizures.

- Androgenic steroids might be prescribed for delayed puberty and hormonal disorders.

- Dehydroepiandrosterone (DHEA) is a hormone used in anti-ageing therapy. It can improve physical performance.

If you are on any of these drugs and develop acne, your doctor will help you solve the problem. Sometimes you can switch to another medication, but it might not always be advisable. Your doctor will help you find a solution for your acne without compromising your health. One possibility is continuing your medication but treating the acne with a different drug.

Please DO NOT stop your medication. The results can be dangerous. You MUST speak to your doctor, who will help you address the acne.

Treatments

Acne is treatable. There is no reason why you have to suffer from acne and its physical and emotional effects. If your acne is mild, start with topical creams you can buy at your pharmacy. If your skin does not improve, get medical help.

If you have tried over-the-counter products without success, it is time to take the next step and get medical advice to end your suffering.

Topical Lotions and Creams

You can buy many topical lotions for acne at your local pharmacy. They are called first-line treatments in the medical world and should help with mild cases of comedones (blackheads and whiteheads) and inflammatory acne. If your acne does not improve dramatically, or worsens, you must see your doctor or dermatologist. They will prescribe a more potent lotion or cream and, in severe cases, possibly oral medication.

First-line/Over-the-Counter Lotions and Creams

Benzoyl peroxide: used for papules and pustules; not used for blackheads and whiteheads. Benzoyl peroxide has been on the market for a long time and is a trusted medication. It kills bacteria in papules. Therefore, doctors often prescribe it with another medicine.

Retinoids: used for blackheads, whiteheads, and papules. Retinoids are the go-to treatment for acne, ageing, and hyperpigmentation. They act as an exfoliator as they remove the dead cells from the very top of your stratum corneum. Retinoids are not a spot treatment; their action is more mechanical. They unclog blocked pores, stimulate the dead cell to shed, and make way for new and healthier cells to come to the outermost skin layer.

This process stimulates new cell formation and lessens pimples and bumps. Although it takes a month for a new cell to reach the surface, several cycles are usually needed for completely healthy cells to form.

There are several versions of retinoids, and your pharmacist or doctor will help you choose the correct retinoid. Speak to a medical professional about the following forms of retinoid:

- Adapalene is a synthetic retinoid with anti-inflammatory properties. Tests have shown it is as effective as tretinoin and less irritating to the skin. If your skin is sensitive, try adapalene.

- Tazarotene, also a retinoid, causes a burning sensation on the skin. Therefore, doctors prescribe it only when less irritating retinoids are not effective.

Azelaic acid: used for blackheads, papules, and rosacea. Azelaic acid is a natural product and a good choice for those trying to stay away from chemicals. It occurs in barley, wheat, and rye and is anti-inflammatory. It destroys the bacteria that cause acne. It is also an antioxidant and thus neutralises harmful free radicals.

If you have acne and hyperpigmentation, azelaic acid is a good first-line topical medication.

Salicylic acid: used for blackheads, papules, and pustules. Salicylic is also a natural product and comes from the bark of the willow tree, but synthetic salicylic acid is also available. It removes dead cells from the skin surface. It also reduces inflammation, and redness and swelling will improve. It is suitable for mild to moderate outbreaks, but severe acne must be treated by a medical professional.

Prescription Topical Creams and Lotions

Tretinoin: Tretinoin contains more potent retinoids than those you can buy over the counter. It is also used for hyperpigmentation treatment. It irritates the skin; consequently, you start with a minimal amount. As your skin gets used to it, the amount is increased.

It increases the rate at which new cells form and thus prevents the pores from clogging. UV radiation destroys retinoids; therefore, you should apply it only at night. Protect your skin with a good sunscreen, as tretinoin thins the stratum corneum, and sunburn and hyperpigmentation are dangers.

Do not use tretinoin and benzoyl peroxide together because of their chemical reaction.

Dapsone: used for inflammatory acne and blackheads. It is also an oral antibiotic. Dapsone is known under a different brand name and is only available with a prescription. It comes in gel form, and you treat the spots with a tiny drop only twice daily.

Dapsone is antimicrobial; it kills the bacteria that cause your acne. It is also an anti-inflammatory and reduces inflamed pimples.

In severe cases of acne, the doctor might prescribe dapsone in combination with benzoyl peroxide. Follow the prescription diligently. Apply one lotion at a time and wait until it is fully absorbed before applying the second one. If these two mix on your skin, your skin will temporarily turn yellow. It can be washed off; still, you don't want to waste time and the product.

When you find retinoids too irritating on your skin, ask your doctor about dapsone. It is a gentler treatment and does not irritate the skin.

Tetracycline: used for inflammatory acne. It is also an oral antibiotic. Tetracycline is used for many bacterial infections and is effective for inflammatory acne. It is only available when prescribed by a doctor. It harms young children and pregnant or nursing women, as the baby will get tetracycline through breastmilk. The doctor will also ensure that your liver and kidney health is good.

You must wear sunscreen when you take tetracycline orally or topically.

Oral Medications

Antibiotics

If you have tried topical medications without any improvement to your acne, your doctor might prescribe an antibiotic for inflammatory acne. Antibiotics attack the bacteria that cause acne.

Follow your doctor's orders carefully when taking antibiotics, especially if they contain tetracycline. Iron and milk decrease the effect of tetracycline; consequently, it is better to take antibiotics on an empty stomach. Furthermore, antibiotics sometimes cause mild gastro problems.

Pregnant women and young children should not take antibiotics containing tetracycline. Speak to your doctor. There are other options available.

Oral antibiotics only show improvements after six to eight weeks. In most cases, you will apply a topical lotion also, as the combination of topical and oral antibiotics is more effective.

Doxycycline is effective for mild and moderate acne but increases the risk of UV radiation. A good sunscreen is necessary and will protect your skin.

Isotretinoin

Isotretinoin is usually a last resort, as it has dangerous side effects. It potentially can cause psychiatric problems and congenital disabilities. Isotretinoin, also known by the brand name Accutane, is a derivative of vitamin A.

Doctors only prescribe isotretinoin for severe cystic or inflammatory acne. Isotretinoin reduces the size of the sebaceous glands; consequently, they produce less sebum. This medication further increases cell shedding and affects the hair follicles. Understandably, reduced sebum, increased cell shedding, and improved hair follicle activities minimise acne.

Dermatologists are hesitant to prescribe isotretinoin for women who might fall pregnant. The danger of birth defects is severe, and women must take two types of birth control while on this medication. They are also not allowed to fall pregnant until at least a month after stopping the drug.

Other side effects are hepatitis, hypertriglyceridemia, intracranial hypertension, arthralgia, myalgias, night blindness, and hyperostosis – although they are rare. Your doctor will also check your liver function every month.

Your doctor will only prescribe isotretinoin if no other treatment works for you. Unfortunately, this dangerous drug is the only medication with a long-term effect.

Birth Control

Some birth control medications can help to reduce acne. It regulates testosterone, which stabilises sebum secretion. You will have to take medicine for an extended period to normalise the hormone levels.

Corticosteroid injections

Doctors only do corticosteroid injections for severe cystic acne that does not respond to other treatments. The specialist injects diluted corticosteroid directly into the cyst. It reduces inflammation and reduces the size of the cyst. It is particularly effective to help prevent scarring.

Mechanical and Laser Light Treatments

Salon Treatments

Salon treatments for acne and hyperpigmentation are similar. It includes facials with salicylic acids, more invasive chemical peels, and laser and light therapy.

These treatments take off the dead cells but also kill inflammation on the skin surface. One session is not enough; you will have to repeat salon visits for several months for the best results.

Chemical peels are effective but even better with simultaneous oral and topical treatments. Consult your dermatologist before starting chemical peels, as they make the skin hypersensitive to UV radiation. Your doctor will warn you if your skin barrier is already too compromised. You could probably go for chemical peels a month after completing the other medications.

You will find more information on these treatments in the chapters on hyperpigmentation and ageing.

Photodynamic Therapy (PDT)

This treatment for severe pustules is not done in a beauty salon but by a qualified dermatologist. The process combines a special topical ingredient with light therapy to destroy inflammation and heal scars and hyperpigmentation.

Avoidance of Trigger Substances

No Squeezing

If your grandmother and mother ever were right, it was when they told you not to squeeze a pimple. Squeezing irritates the skin and infects the acne spot and the surrounding area. Worse still, it can cause long-term scarring and hyperpigmentation.

Sunburn

Many topical lotions, orally taken medications, and salon treatments weaken the skin barrier and make the skin more susceptible to UV radiation. Retinoids, for example, act as an exfoliate and take off the topmost cells of the stratum corneum. Consequently, your skin is much more fragile, and the sun can damage your skin badly. You might end up with unsightly hyperpigmentation on top of acne.

Very importantly, you might get skin cancer if your skin is not protected from UV radiation during treatment. Be careful, and never leave the house without a good sunscreen.

Quick Reminder

There is no such thing as flawless skin. Some people only hide their flaws better than others.

Our imperfections add to our unique beauty. However, when your flaw threatens your self-esteem and your skin causes embarrassment, seek help immediately.

There are two types of acne: comedones and inflammatory acne.

Comedones are blackheads and whiteheads.

Inflammatory acne is papules, pustules, nodal, and cystic lumps.

You can treat mild and moderate acne with over-the-counter products.

Only a medical doctor can treat severe acne.

Chapter 7:
Electrolysis – Answer to Unwanted Hair

Beauty is the promise of happiness.

If you are ever in doubt about what beauty is, read Edmund Burke's book *A Philosophical Enquiry into the Origin of Our Ideas of the Sublime and Beautiful*. If philosophy is not your cup of tea, at least take this clever 18th-century statesman, economist, and philosopher's words to heart if you struggle with unwanted facial hair: Beauty is the promise of happiness.

This chapter helps you understand where unwanted hair comes from and how to remove it permanently. Its aim is to tell you everything about electrolysis and help you overcome your reservations about the process.

Unwanted hair can be permanently removed. It is not something one can say unequivocally about any other skin condition. Therefore, it is worth repeating. It is possible to remove unwanted hair forever with electrolysis.

Research in the 21st Century

Experiments with electrolysis started already in the late 19th century with good results. (Chapter 15 explains all about the exciting history of hair removal.) However, researchers only recently discovered the complexity of the bulb at the bottom of the hair follicle. They also realised that by killing the heart of the bulb, they could stop the hair from growing again.

The 'Bulge' Discovery

In the 21st century, scientists returned to the life cycle of the hair follicle. Until the early 2000s, biologists believed stem cells originated from the bulb. The bulb at the bottom of the hair follicle consists of the matrix cells (which will not be discussed here) and the dermal papilla. New research proved that the stem cells are in the bulge at the opening of the sebaceous gland and the outer root sheath, not in the bulb.

These stem cells proliferate and regenerate the hair follicles, the sebaceous glands, and the epidermis. It is an exciting science that has since played a vital role in treating hair disorders. It also contributed to the development of more effective hair care products.

Very important for women struggling with unwanted hair, it became clear why electrolysis is so successful in destroying the hair follicle permanently. During the growth phase (anagen), the follicle lengthens downward. The stem cells in the bulge multiply and push the dermal papilla downward also. Thus the current released during electrolysis kills the stem cells and blood flow to the follicle. It ensures that regrowth cannot take place.

Body Hair and Health: Causes of Unwanted Hair

Frida Kahlo is still famous nearly 70 years after her death. Her self-portraits decorate everything from walls to tea cloths. Her most recognisable feature was not her limp but her monobrow. According to legend, she used an eyebrow pencil to accentuate her unique beauty feature.

Despite Frida loving her brows and using them to enhance her beauty, many women pluck a few unwanted hairs regularly. Electrolysis is suitable for all hair types, whether for a few stray hairs on the chin or too much fuzz on your legs.

Electrolysis dramatically improves the lives of women with male-pattern hair growth (Hirsutism), as well as transgender and non-binary people. Electrolysis is a lifesaver for them.

What Is Normal Hair Growth?

Not all women are equal in this regard, and some ethnic groups have more body hair than others. People from the Middle East, Mediterranean, Mexico, Puerto Rico, Cuba, Central and South America, and Spanish cultures often have strong hair growth. Women with thin hair often envy their lovely hairdos, forgetting that these women might not be happy with their body hair.

The Ferriman-Gallwey scale measures hair growth on body sites that could show signs of unbalanced androgens. This scale considers ethnicity and does not add a specific number to 'what is normal'. Doctors find this scientific method helpful in establishing whether a woman needs treatment for male-patterned hair growth.

There are several options:

- If insulin-resistant, a healthy diet and weight management can make a difference.

- Oral contraceptives are also effective.

- If needed, emotional support will be given.

There is no reason to live with unwanted hair. You can get medical treatment and electrolysis at the same time.

Types of Hair

During their lifetime, humans have three types of hair:

- Lanugo hair is the soft, thin hair that covers a newborn baby. These hairs are usually unpigmented and found all over the body except for the lips, genitals, palms, and soles of the feet. Lanugo hair is short and does not have a medulla – an innermost layer of thicker hair comprised of cells and air spaces. These baby hairs disappear within two months after birth.

- Vellus hair is soft and often called peach fuzz. It covers most of the body in both male and female children, but the length and colour differ in individuals. They help to regulate temperature and play an important role in touch.

- Terminal hair starts during puberty and replaces some vellus hair. They are longer, coarser, and pigmented, presenting as dark or even black hair on the face and body. There are three distinct groups of terminal hair:

  Asexual hair is already present at birth in both male and female babies. Growth hormones stimulate asexual hair growth. It is on the scalp, eyebrows, eyelashes, forearms, and legs.

  Ambisexual hair appears in both sexes during puberty, stimulated by steroid hormone production. These hairs are found in the armpit, pubis, lower limbs, and abdomen. Ambisexual hair growth differs from person to person and also between the sexes.

Sexual hair is stimulated by androgen production and found in the nasal passages, moustache, the back, and chest. Sexual hair is usually more profound in people defined as male at birth, as they have higher testosterone levels.

Polycystic Ovary Syndrome (PCOS)

If you have Polycystic Ovary Syndrome, your body produces too many male hormones. It causes weight gain and prevents ovulation and acne. Unfortunately, Polycystic Ovary Syndrome also affects the hair: Male-pattern hair develops on the face and body, and hair growth on the scalp thins, similar to male baldness.

Polycystic Ovary Syndrome is the most common cause of Hirsutism.

It usually starts around the time of the first menstruation and often occurs in people with obesity. Symptoms are irregular periods, excess androgens, and Hirsutism. Doctors also attributed Polycystic Ovary Syndrome to excess insulin, low-grade inflammation, and genetic propensity.

Hirsutism (Male-Patterned Hair Growth)

Hirsutism is a recognised disease but carries a dark history of being strange and abnormal. Many travelling circuses featured a bearded lady in their freak shows for centuries. It was beyond cruel, and one can only imagine the emotional turmoil these poor women had to suffer every day of their lives. Often rejected by their families, they became outcasts and had no other way to survive.

Hirsutism is the condition where a woman's facial hair resembles a man's. But what does it mean? Do you have Hirsutism when you have a few coarse hairs around the chin?

Remember, all genders have male hormones (androgens), and a few persistent unwelcome hairs do not mean your hormones are unbalanced. However, if you experience a sudden increase in hair growth, consider the following before you panic or rush off to your doctor.

Male-patterned hair growth refers to the hair above the belly button, the chest, upper back, and face. A few hairs around your nipples are normal. If you have more than eight hairs around a nipple, or the hair on your head is thinning, similar to male baldness, your hormones might be unbalanced. It means your oestrogen levels are declining, and your testosterone levels are rising (Gorman, 2020).

Do not self-diagnose or despair. See your doctor about the possibility of Hirsutism. Medical treatment is available; you do not have to live with the embarrassment of a beard or chest hair.

Transwomen

Gender terminology is complicated, and rightly so. We are humans with varying gender identifications. Thankfully, we live in a time when the right to be unique is officially respected. However, people uneasy with the sex allocated to them at birth, which clashes with their inner identity, still experience prejudice.

Fortunately, medical, psychological, and aesthetical procedures are available to accompany transgender people on this challenging road. A multi-disciplinary approach is followed:

Psychologists help with emotional issues and work with the person to improve self-esteem, body well-being, and quality of life. Psychologists involve family members and help them understand that transgender is not an illness but the desire to match the body with the true identity.

Electrolysis helps to remove facial and body hair permanently. It often is a lifeline to transgender women, as it improves their appearance dramatically. Electrolysis often goes hand in hand with feminising hormone therapy.

Medical treatment is a long and complicated process not discussed in this book. Because hormones play a vital role in male-pattern hair growth, we will briefly touch on gene-affirming hormone therapy. Your doctor and psychologist will guide you through this process. Nonetheless, basic information will prepare you ahead of your appointments.

Feminising Hormone Therapy

A transgender woman takes feminising hormones to help change the body into a more feminine shape. Breasts develop, the skin becomes softer, the testicles shrink, and the hips gradually become rounder.

Transgender males take masculinising hormones to block menstruation, promote male-pattern hair growth, form muscles, and deepen the voice. Feminising and masculinising hormones are called gender-affirming hormone therapy.

Transgender women often receive feminine hormones together with a blocker for masculine hormones. In general, feminising hormone therapy is very effective and a tremendous help in changing the biological gender.

In many cases, feminising hormone therapy does not stop unwanted hair growth entirely. However, a combination of hormone treatment and electrolysis destroys hair growth effectively.

What Is Electrolysis?

Electrolysis is a hair removal treatment that destroys the hair root. It is the only permanent method to remove hair from the face and body.

Electrolysis Methods

Three methods of electrolysis have been used since its discovery:

- *Short-wave diathermy (thermolysis)* is an alternating current created from the vibration of the cells.

- *The galvanic* method chemically destroys the follicle.

- The *blend* combines both methods; heat speeding up the galvanic chemical reaction to destroy the follicle.

Process

Modern electrolysis machines are computerised. These hi-tech machines process information precisely and smoothly without interruption. It gives the electrologist the advantage of precisely and accurately controlling the current intensity and timing.

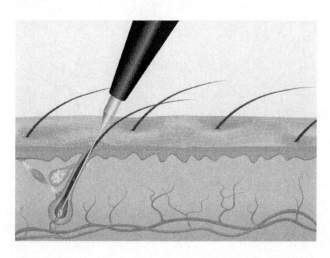

A certified technician inserts a fine, sterile probe, the same diameter as a hair, into the hair follicle. A small, controlled amount of energy – an electrical current – is then discharged into the follicle. The follicle is destroyed by one of the three methods discussed above.

Most clients have repeated treatments every ten days until the hair growth slows down. The treatment causes the hair to become weaker and slower to reappear. The time between treatments gets longer as hair growth slackens.

Hair grows in cycles, and the individual hair is destroyed during the growth (anagen) phase. The dermal papilla supplying the blood to the hair follicle is weakest as the hair shaft just appears on the surface. It is most effective to have the treatment during the growth phase, as the current can destroy the stem cells and blood flow, thus killing the hair follicle.

Hair Growth Cycles

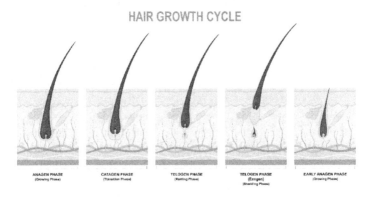

Anagen Phase (Growing Phase) • Catagen Phase (Transition Phase) • Telogen Phase (Resting Phase) • Telogen Phase (Exogen) (Shedding Phase) • Early Anagen Phase (Growing Phase)

Anagen: Growth Stage

You might wonder what the chances are of getting this timing right. The good news is that 90% of the hair is in the growth phase at any given time. The growth phase lasts up to seven years on the scalp (Stocum, 2013). Your eyebrows, lashes, and body hair have a shorter growth cycle.

The bottom line is that most electrolysis probes will reach their target and be successful. The matrix cells are constantly supplied with fresh oxygen-rich blood. Consequently, they actively divide and form a new hair sheath from where the new hair grows.

Catagen: Transitional Stage

During this very short, roughly two-week transition, the hair bulb at the bottom of the follicle separates from the dermal papilla and moves upward toward the sebaceous gland. The bulb and the lower follicle start to disintegrate.

Telogen: Resting Stage

During the rest period, the hair remains close to the sebaceous gland until it sheds naturally. The length of the resting stage differs for different types of hair. The thicker and somewhat coarser hair of the eyebrows and lashes (terminal hair) rest between three to four months. The much thinner and fine body hair (vellus hair) rests for a shorter period, around two and a half months.

Exogen: Shedding Stage

Humans lose their hair naturally over a period of time; fortunately, not all at the same time. The synchronised way in which the body sheds hair confirms the wonder of the human body. Between 80 to 90% of your hair is always in the anagen stage; thus, you will always have the majority of your hair (Sampson, 2019.

If the hair is deliberately plucked from the hair follicle outside this natural cycle, as in waxing, the growth cycle will be stimulated, thus delaying the electrolysis treatment.

Keeping the natural hair growth cycle in mind, it is understandable that electrolysis is a complicated and precise process and explains why repeated sessions are necessary. Most women have sessions at ten-day intervals, and it can take between 18 and 254 months to destroy all the unwanted hair follicles.

Preparation for Electrolysis

So, you have decided and are about to start your exciting beauty journey! For most people, it is a big step. You probably have been on an emotional rollercoaster: excitement and doubt simultaneously. You might even have felt exposed and embarrassed during the consultation. Be assured that your technician has been trained to assist you on this journey.

Never lose sight of why you embarked on this journey. You want to remove unwanted hair because these hairs make you unhappy and prevent you from being the woman you are deep inside. Remember, you are not doing this for other people. This journey is for you and your quality of life.

How do you prepare?

Before Consultation

- Stop using all retinol products and alpha-hydroxy acids – (AHAs) and synthetic alpha-hydroxy acids (BHAs) – two weeks before your consultation, as they make the skin sensitive and fragile.

- Also, stop all short-term hair removal a week before your consultation so the technician can better assess the area and discuss a treatment plan.

- During your consultation and before the treatment, your technician will discuss pain medications and topical numbing agents that you can take ahead of your session.

Before and Between Treatments

- Stop all short-term hair removal a week before your treatment, as the hairs must begin to re-emerge to allow more hairs to be removed.

- No tweezing, plucking, or waxing between sessions. They remove the hair root and will slow down the electrolysis process.

- On treatment day, do not use any creams or deodorants on the area that will be treated.

- Drink lots of water ahead of your appointments. You must stay well hydrated.

Care After Electrolysis

Take care of yourself emotionally by staying positive. Electrolysis is a slow process, but the results are everlasting. Temporary inconveniences pass soon enough: Your future with smooth skin is at stake. Patience is the key, so keep the end goal in sight.

Be prepared for your skin to be swollen for a day or two. It is usually worse for people with sensitive skin. It is perfectly normal and will disappear soon enough.

Katie Lewis, the book's co-author, is a British Institute of Electrolysis member. She insists that 50% of the treatment is in aftercare. During the procedure, moisture is taken from the hair follicle and must be replaced. Apply a hydrating moisturiser twice a day. Katie recommends aloe vera during the first 24 hours of treatment. Also, use sunscreen with SPF 50 to avoid hyperpigmentation.

If any symptoms persist, contact your technician.

- Plan ahead and have a meal or two in the freezer so you don't have to go out if you don't feel like it.

- Line up a good book or a movie to keep your mind off your skin.

- Use the after-care product the technician will provide. It will calm any irritability soon enough.

- Don't use any other creams or lotions on the treated area.

- Small brown scabs might appear, especially in areas where body hairs were distorted or ingrowing. They are your skin's way of naturally healing the minute wounds obtained during electrolysis. Don't pick them: They will fall off within a day or two.

- Stay out of the sun, heated areas, saunas, or any place where you will sweat excessively.

- It is best not to do intense exercises for two days after treatment.

- Don't touch your face: It can cause infection.

Find a Certified Technician

Your choice of an electrolysis technician is vital. Electrolysis is a highly specialised field. In the United Kingdom, technicians must hold Level 3 anatomy and physiology. They also must have an accredited beauty therapy certificate or a nursing qualification. Companies providing electrolysis machines do extensive in-house training.

Most countries require electrolysis technicians to register at a certification board. They have to renew their licences annually, and their premises are also inspected regularly to ensure patient safety from the spreading of skin infections.

Visit the salon if you are considering electrolysis. If you aren't confident to directly ask, go for another treatment such as waxing and meet the staff. You will get a good idea of general cleanliness, but especially of the attitude and care you can expect.

Also, ask about qualifications or read the certificates that are displayed. Check for dates to see whether they are fully updated.

Electrolysis is entirely safe in the hands of a qualified technician. Most countries in the world regulate electrolysis practices. A short summary of the different authorities follows below.

Global Legislation in a Nutshell

Australia

Under the Public Health Act, electrolysis technicians must register and obtain certification and a licence to operate in Australia. They must follow strict health and safety guidelines. Local councils administer the licencing.

Canada

Electrologists must have a certified qualification from an accredited training institute. The Federation of Canadian Electrolysis Association coordinates education and registration to ensure the highest standards. Practising electrologists must have provincial membership. The Federation offers continuous training opportunities to keep up with developments in the field and ensure safety.

European Union

UNI-Europa Hair & Beauty represents 17 trade unions in 13 countries (Uni Europa Hair & Beauty, n.d.). Understandably, the legislation differs from country to country. Wherever you live, research the training and certification of electrolysis technicians and only trust a fully licenced and certified professional.

New Zealand

The New Zealand Association of Registered Beauty Therapists ensures that international standards are followed. Therapists must have a national certificate to practice and a licence from local councils. An environmental health inspector checks the premises annually to ensure hygiene and health regulations are strictly executed.

United Kingdom

Electrolysis in the U.K. falls under the Local Government (Miscellaneous Provisions) Act 1982. Premises are inspected annually. The technician must display a valid copy of their licence at all times.

United States of America

The American Food and Drug Administration (FDA) approved electrolysis as the only permanent hair removal method. The various states in the USA regulate electrolysis, and some rules and regulations might differ from state to state. Valid licences are usually required.

Furthermore, American training institutions are accredited by the National Accrediting Commission of Career Arts & Science, Accrediting Commission of Career Schools and Colleges, or the Council of Occupational Education. These institutions ensure that electrolysis technicians are trained to the highest standards.

Laser Removal for Unwanted Hair: Reduction Only

What Is Laser Hair Removal?

Despite what you may read in online advertisements, laser therapy does not remove hair permanently. A google search on permanent hair removal will tell you differently, and many people are misled in this way. There are numerous sites promoting laser removal for unwanted hair. It is always wise to check who promotes a product: When a company or individual sells a specific product, they will, of course, emphasise the positives.

At most, laser removal is a hair reduction method only. A light beam emits concentrated light to the follicle. Melanin, the colour pigment in hair, absorbs the light and converts the light into heat. The heat damages the hair follicle and slows down future hair growth.

Unfortunately, even multiple laser treatments do not stop regrowth permanently. Regular maintenance treatments are needed.

Interestingly, a laser works best on people with light skin and dark hair. Dark hair has more melanin, which absorbs the light beams. Lighter skin has less melanin and is thus not affected by the laser.

Unfortunately, people with little contrast between hair and skin colour are more at risk. The laser should target the melanin in the hair, not the skin. A laser may damage dark skin, sometimes only temporarily. In severe cases, the skin might be pigmented permanently.

Several treatments are necessary, usually no more than six, with an interval of approximately eight weeks between treatments. The patient wears special glasses to protect the eyes. Your doctor will apply a topical numbing cream. Some lasers have a cooling device at the tip; alternatively, the doctor applies a cooling gel.

A small area like the upper lip is treated in a few minutes, but a big area like the back will take much longer. The hairs do not shed immediately but gradually fall out over the next few days.

Your skin will be slightly red and irritated. Ice helps to soothe the burning sensation.

Quick Questions

What is the difference between laser and electrolysis?

Laser technology treats large areas simultaneously. Hair growth slows down but does not stop permanently. Laser therapy is a hair reduction only.

Electrolysis is the only proven permanent hair removal system globally verified by health authorities. Electrolysis treats each hair follicle separately and destroys each one permanently.

Is electrolysis safe?

Electrolysis is entirely safe if done by a certified technician who is appropriately qualified. Your technician will assist you during the preparation and aftercare phases.

Does electrolysis remove hair permanently?

Yes, it is the only permanent hair removal method. Health authorities approve it in most countries.

What types of electrolysis are there?

There are three types: galvanic (chemical), thermolysis (localised heat), and the blend method. The blend method uses a combination of thermolysis and galvanic techniques.

How long is the treatment?

A treatment every ten days allows the skin to recover fully. The length and number of treatments vary from person to person, as each client has a different hair growth density. It is impossible to give the exact number of treatments, but allow between 18 to 24 months. During the last phase, you will need fewer treatments as hair growth slows down, and the intervals between sessions will become longer.

I am afraid of needles; will I be alright?

The British Institute and Association of Electrolysis (BIAE) prefers to use the term 'probe'. The tiny probe is the same size as an eyelash, just about visible to the naked eye. It enters the natural opening of the hair follicle, and you will not feel anything.

Does it hurt?

Electrolysis machines have come a long way to make the process comfortable for the client, though they do not eradicate all sensation. When the current is applied, you will feel a hot sensation. The technician applies a numbing cream to minimise this.

I am a blood donor; can I still have electrolysis?

You must stop donating blood until a few months after your last session. It is a precaution to prevent the transfer of any possible viruses or bacteria.

How do I prepare for treatment?

Stop using all retinol treatments two weeks before your appointment. Also, do not use any short-term hair removal for the week before treatment (shaving, waxing, plucking, etc.).

What can go wrong?

The risks are minimal if done by a certified technician; at most, slight skin reddening.

What must be avoided?

Exercise, sauna, steam, swimming, sunbathing, sunbeds, make-up, scented products, and do not touch the area.

Will I be scarred?

Scarring is most unlikely if done by a certified technician. People with darker skin might have temporary dark spots, but they fade over time. Do not use lightening creams during electrolysis.

How soon can I go back to work after a session?

You can return to work the following day, but you *must* follow the technician's instructions 100%.

Chapter 8:
Premature Ageing Can Be Managed

There is no definition of beauty, but when you can see someone's spirit coming through, something unexplainable, that's beautiful.

Most women have a sense of what the actress Liv Tyler meant with the words above. But most women will struggle to explain it, as Ms. Tyler admitted. Maybe it helps to eliminate what ageing beauty is not: It is not trying to look younger.

So often, ageing women resort to heavy make-up to cover up the marks of time. Unfortunately, layers of foundation and carefully drawn lines around the eyes have the opposite effect: You don't look younger; you look tired, hard, and unnatural.

Your appearance and skincare reflect something of your personality, hygiene, state of mind, and spirit. Maybe enduring beauty is looking for the best version of yourself at any age. And the best version of oneself at any age − young or old − boils down to being well-kept.

Sadly, some women give up on their appearance somewhere along the line, accepting the signs of ageing as inevitable. They usually proudly announce that their beauty routine consists of soap and water. It is as if they defiantly say to the world: Take me as I am.

Does it mean you must accept dry skin, greying hair, and sagging jowls? Natural beauty is not carelessness or self-neglect: An attractive older woman's face and body language radiate self-acceptance and peace. Liv Tyler's 'unexplained beauty' might mean that a woman reflects inner strength and happiness even though life has thrown her a few curveballs.

Ageing gracefully does not necessarily equal expensive creams and salon treatments. These are a bonus if you can afford them. But there is an element of graceful ageing that cannot be found in creams or salons, and that is inner peace.

For many years, people accepted that physical decline, disease, and disappearing looks inevitably go along with ageing. Modern science helps people live longer and have a quality of life for much longer. The next chapter explains how lifestyle choices, diet, healthy living, exercise, happiness, and avoidance of UV radiation and pollution can add to skin quality and appearance. We now know beauty is not only about what you put on your face but also how you treat your body and your soul.

Your skin is what the world sees. It speaks much louder than your words: It reveals your health, how much you care, and even divulges your private sins, such as smoking, excessive alcohol, or sunbathing.

But it is never too late. You cannot change the past, but you can improve the quality of your skin by caring for it now. This chapter deals with the ageing skin – the internal and external causes. Also, we will see how you can make the best of your skin and be the best version of yourself, whatever your age.

Skin Ageing Is Complex

The first chapter discusses the structure of the skin and how it functions. This chapter builds on that and discusses the *processes in the skin*, especially those that cause skin ageing. Skin ageing is a complex process: Firstly, you age because of the natural deterioration of the skin itself, and secondly, external factors damage the skin even more. Chapter 10 discusses the external factors contributing to skin ageing in more detail.

The skin is damaged from the inside and outside. These intrinsic changes and extrinsic damage do not happen overnight. It builds up over the years. Initially, one scarcely notices the changes, but in the end, natural ageing and external damage catch up with you.

So when is the skin aged, dry, or only dehydrated? Dry skin lacks oil; dehydrated skin lacks water.

You can do a quick test on the back of your hand to test whether your skin is dehydrated. Pinch the skin and let go. If it returns to normal immediately, your skin is probably dry and needs moisturising. However, if the skin takes longer than three seconds to return to normal, your skin is dehydrated. Drink plenty of fluids and avoid heat and sweating.

Visible Signs of Ageing Skin

- Healing takes longer.

- Hair follicles become less active, and hair thins.

- Natural fat levels in the skin change and redistribute.

- The epidermis gets drier as the sebaceous glands produce less sebum.

- There are fewer melanocytes in the epidermis, and the skin pales and is less resistant to UV radiation.

- The dermis sags as less collagen is formed.

- Sweat gland activity reduces, and heat becomes a problem.

- Blood supply to the dermis is reduced.

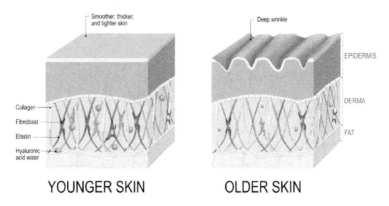

YOUNGER SKIN   OLDER SKIN

Intrinsic Factors Causing Ageing Skin

Aged skin is usually attributed to changes in the stratum corneum, but the real cause lies deeper: damage within the cells and the stem cells' inability to repair the damage. Furthermore, gravity takes its toll: Muscles weaken, bone decreases, and fat diminishes and moves to change your features. As the skin sags, the shape and contours of the face change.

Aged skin is thin with little elasticity. Cell rejuvenation declines as cellular turnover in the epidermis slows down. Thus, new cells take much longer to move to the epidermis, and dead corneocytes' shedding becomes slower.

The rate at which intrinsic or chronological ageing happens depends on general health, personal care, and ethnicity. From the information in the chapter on ethnic beauty, we know that women with dark skin show signs of ageing much later than women with light skin.

Stratum Corneum and Ageing

It might be paper-thin and consists primarily of dead corneocytes, but the stratum corneum is intricately put together. Its ability to hold different types of natural moisturisers makes it difficult to believe that the stratum corneum primarily comprises dead cells.

Ageing skin has a dull colour and a rough texture with ridges because of low moisture levels in the stratum corneum. With age, the stratum corneum's ability to maintain natural moisturisers decreases.

Still, a lot is going on in this outermost layer of the skin. The stratum corneum consists mainly of ceramides, fatty acids, and cholesterol. It has a natural moisturising factor, which dermatologists refer to as NMF. The natural moisturising factor is a mixture of water-soluble compounds. Furthermore, it contains lipids, sebum, and aquaporin. Some researchers say the stratum corneum also contains hyaluronic acid (Sakai, 2000).

To refresh your mind:

- Lipids are natural oils.

- The sebaceous gland secretes sebum through the hair follicle. Sebum is a natural moisturiser.

- Hyaluronic acid is a humectant that can hold up to 1,000 times its size in water.

- Aquaporin is a protein found in the cell membranes that lets water through.

- Ceramides are natural oily wax with strings of amino acids (which form proteins) attached.

- Fatty acids are the building blocks of the natural fat in our bodies. They appear in groups of three, and these groups are called triglycerides.

- Epidermal cholesterol is a type of lipid, thus a natural moisturiser.

- Corneocytes are dead keratinocytes and make up most of the stratum corneum.

You might wonder what cholesterol is doing to your skin. Cholesterol, ceramides, and fatty acids together form the skin barrier. They help retain water and the skin's natural moisturisers in the stratum corneum. They also protect the skin from germs entering, as they form a shield on the surface.

When the skin barrier is intact with plenty of natural moisturisers in the corneum stratum, the skin looks fresh and hydrated. However, when the skin barrier is damaged and the natural moisturisers are lost, the skin is more susceptible to damage from outside.

Transepidermal Water Loss (TEWL) and Ageing

Dermatologists call moisture loss in the epidermis transepidermal water loss (TEWL). A balanced stratum corneum, with no damage, retains moisture. When the stratum corneum is damaged, the skin is dry and more prone to further harm.

Moisture loss also affects the enzymes in the cell junction membranes – desmosomes. The desmosomes don't function properly without moisture. Dead cell shedding, or desquamation, is slower, and corneocytes (dead keratinocytes) accumulate on the skin surface. They cause a dull, rough, and dry texture.

Damage from the Outside

It has been said numerous times that UV radiation – sunburn – is the worst thing you can do to your skin. Harsh chemicals in soaps and lotions also damage the stratum corneum. Thus, go slow on acetone, chlorine, and detergents. Also, don't stay too long in the water. It dehydrates the skin. Poor eating habits, too much alcohol, and a lack of sleep damage your skin and health as well.

Dermo-Epidermal Junction's Role in Ageing

A membrane between the epidermis and the dermis holds the epidermis and the dermis together. It consists primarily of keratinocytes and is enriched by dermal fibroblasts. The epidermis has no blood vessels and gets nutrients from the dermis through the porous junction membrane. With age, the dermo-epidermal membrane separates slowly; consequently, fewer nutrients reach the epidermis.

Dermis Structure Role in Ageing

In the nucleus, the centre of each cell is a chromosome. Experts believe cellular ageing is connected to the little caps that protect the ends of these chromosomes. These caps are called telomeres; with age, they shorten and fail to protect the chromosome and the cell's recycling ability.

Decreased Collagen and Ageing

The dermis comprises an extracellular matrix, a strong mesh of collagen and elastin cells. The matrix gives structure to and supports the skin.

Collagen is the primary protein in the skin. As we age, less collagen is formed. In young skin, the collagen is neatly organised in fibre bundles, but in older skin, collagen is irregular and fragmented. It does not bind with elastin as effectively as in young skin.

Fibroblasts' Function and Ageing

Fibroblasts are connective tissue that is responsible for cell rejuvenation. Enzymes in older skin break down fibroblasts.

Fibroblasts produce collagen but also stimulate donor cells to form new cells. Therefore, the effect on the skin is significant when fibroblast function is slowed down by chronological ageing or external damage. The skin's internal balance is disturbed, less collagen is produced, and skin renewal slows down. It causes loss of elasticity, wrinkling, and pigmentation. In short, the skin loses its glow and becomes dull and rough.

Decreased Elastin and Ageing

During one's 30s and 40s, natural elastin production starts to decrease. Furthermore, smoking, alcohol, unhealthy eating patterns, and a lack of exercise break down elastin. The bad news is elastin cannot be replenished by any oral or topical compound.

Although you can't replenish elastin, you can prevent accelerated breakdown by living healthily. Inflammation breaks down collagen and elastin; consequently, targeting chronic inflammation will affect the reduction of these two vital proteins in the skin. Read more about chronic inflammation later in this chapter.

The Hypodermis, or Subcutaneous Fat Layer, and Ageing

The hypodermis, the natural fat layer at the bottom of the skin, connects the skin with the bones and muscles, supports the face, and gives form to your face. The fresh layer of fat adding dimension to the cheekbones seems to disappear over time. In its place, the lower face becomes heavy with hanging jowls.

The effect on the upper face becomes visible as facial fats disappear from the middle and upper parts. The eyelids droop, and under-eye bags form. The folds next to the nose are deeper, and the nose tip may also droop. Wrinkles form and the eyes look sunken and hollow. The lips lose volume and become thinner. The worst might be the corners of the mouth, which turn downward as if one is eternally disgusted with life.

In some people, the fat patches do not distribute symmetrically, and they develop asymmetrical features.

It is not a pretty picture, but dermal fillers can efficiently address this aspect of ageing. Dermal fillers consist primarily of hyaluronic acid, a natural compound in your skin. Additionally, dermal fillers work instantly and restore volume instantly. Your doctor can also inject dermal fillers to restore deeper fat pads and thus restore form and structure to the face.

Dermal fillers are costly, but they last up to 18 months and have few side effects.

Hormones, Menopause, and Ageing

Hormones are the body's secret agents. They work behind the scenes to synchronise our biological processes and form part of the endocrine system.

The endocrine system is made up of glands that produce hormones. These glands are distributed across the body: the hypothalamus, pineal, and pituitary glands in the brain, the thyroid in the neck, the adrenals on the kidneys, the pancreas, and the ovaries in the pelvis.

New research has identified the skin as part of the endocrine system. Scientists say the skin reacts to hormones' messages and produces enzymes. Though the skin is part of the body's endocrine system, the skin also produces some hormones. Therefore, it is understandable that a reduction in hormones will worsen skin quality. Unfortunately, when hormone production slows down, the skin ages.

The body has more than 50 hormones (EPA, 2022); some significantly affect the skin and hair during menopause. The blood carries the hormones to various destinations in the body, where special receptors receive the hormones' messages.

Hormones control the body's biological processes. They influence nearly all aspects of our health, immune system, inflammation, sexual health, skin repair, and cellular growth. Hormonal imbalance can cause several diseases, some of which are discussed in previous chapters, including Polycystic Ovary Syndrome and acne. Others include irregular menstruation, infertility, and diabetes type 2.

This section concentrates on hormones' role in skin health and their contribution to skin ageing: dryness, coarseness, thinning, skin tags, and dark skin in the armpit or around the neck area.

Menopause and Hormones

On average, menopause sets in at age 51, but some women can start decades earlier. Menopause continues for two to five years, depending on several environmental factors (Zouboullis, 2022). During menopause, the body goes through significant hormonal changes; especially the sex hormones, oestrogen, and testosterone decrease dramatically.

During the first five years of menopause, collagen production decreases by 30%, and the skin becomes thinner (Zouboullis, 2022).

Hormones are intricate and complex chemicals. If you sense a hormonal imbalance during menopause, speak to a doctor. Do not self-diagnose; it is not something you can tackle on your own. What works for your neighbour will not necessarily work for you. Usually, a simple blood test will identify the problem. Your doctor or an endocrinologist is qualified to advise you.

Oestrogen, the Female Hormone

Oestrogen is known as the female sex hormone, produced by the ovaries and the adrenal glands. Natural oestrogen declines during menopause, but external factors like stress, sleep disruption, and poor diet impact the adrenal glands' function even further.

Oestrogen is a tricky hormone that significantly impacts the body and is invaluable for skin health. It boosts natural collagen, elastin, and hyaluronic acid production. Fortunately, one can replenish oestrogen to maintain the skin's collagen and elasticity. Oestrogen application improves skin thickness and the skin's ability to retain moisture.

Diet can play a vital role in stimulating natural oestrogens, and the next chapter will tell more about foods good for oestrogen.

Testosterone, Not Only a Male Hormone

Testosterone is the male hormone, but healthy women need limited testosterone levels for good general health. It plays a role in forming new red blood cells and maintaining sexual drive and muscle strength.

However, unbalanced levels of testosterone can cause acne. Women with too high levels of testosterone also have dry skin. Other symptoms are frontal balding, increased muscle mass, and a deepening voice.

Interestingly, some women have too low testosterone levels. For them, the doctor might prescribe hormone replacement therapy with a low dose of testosterone.

Dehydroepiandrosterone (DHEA), the 'Mother' of Sex Hormones

Dehydroepiandrosterone (DHEA) is produced by the adrenal glands, and its long name indicates the hormone's complexity. Think of DHEA as a mother hormone delivering the other sex hormones as it helps produce oestrogen and testosterone. It is abundant in youth and gradually declines with age.

Many experts recommend oral and topical DHEA treatments for ageing skin. Topical creams improve brightness and reduce dryness. It also stimulates sebum production and surface hydration.

It is regularly prescribed, but note that too high doses can have severe side effects. It might cause excessively oily skin, acne, increased hair growth, and breast tenderness. Once again, do not self-diagnose. Speak to a medical professional.

Insulin and Collagen Production

Usually, when we refer to insulin, we think of blood sugar, diabetes, overweight, and obesity. Recent research links higher than normal insulin in the body to skin tags and several other serious skin diseases. Multiple skin tags might even be a warning of unknown diabetes type 2.

But insulin affects more than diabetes. Researchers at Brown University linked low insulin levels to longevity (Brown University, 2004).

However, too high levels of insulin also cause ageing. When insulin levels drop, collagen production is reduced.

Insulin and testosterone also play a role in Polycystic Ovary Syndrome, contributing to acne and Hirsutism.

Cortisol, the Brain, and the Skin

When stressed, the body goes into fight-or-flight mode and releases cortisol to prepare the muscles for action. Stress, anxiety, and depression are both in the mind and the body: Stress triggers the adrenal glands that release cortisol. Cortisol causes several physiological processes in the body: The heart rate accelerates, the breathing quickens, the muscles tighten, and the blood pressure rises.

The skin is also affected by cortisol. It stimulates the sebaceous glands to produce more sebum, clog pores, and cause acne. Cortisol also affects the immune system, which can cause sensitivity, redness, and even hives. Furthermore, excess cortisol worsens skin conditions like eczema, psoriasis, and rosacea.

Chronic stress has a prolonged negative effect on skin health. One cannot always control stress levels but should manage them to the best of one's ability. Seek counselling or investigate meditation, mindfulness, or yoga. These are not pie-in-the-sky solutions but are very effective for stress relief.

Melatonin, Not Only a Sleep Hormone

Melatonin should not be confused with melanin, the colour pigment in the skin. The names sound similar, but they are not related.

For many years, melatonin and serotonin were regarded as sleep hormones. It regulates the circadian (day-and-night) rhythm as well as seasonal biorhythms. Formerly appreciated mostly for its role in sleep patterns, melatonin is now known to help control body weight and boost immunity.

Over the last decades, scientists have discovered that melatonin is vital for skin health. The pea-sized pineal gland in the brain is the main source of melatonin. But the skin also produces some melatonin in the keratinocytes, melanocytes, and different parts of the hair follicle. Experts now rate melatonin as a major antioxidant. Its chemical formula interacts with several free radicals and prevents damage to the keratinocytes in the skin.

Nowadays, melatonin is a potent ingredient in many skincare products. Experts recommend that melatonin be applied topically, as it can penetrate the stratum corneum (Klesxcynski, 2012). Oral supplements of melatonin are not equally successful, though. The liver degrades melatonin and prevents sufficient amounts of melatonin from reaching the skin.

Progesterone, the Glow of Pregnancy

Progesterone levels start to decline in the 30s, resulting in dull skin. Interestingly, pregnant women have high levels of progesterone, which cause the glow we attribute to the joy of having a baby. Progesterone is good for skin elasticity and improves blood flow to the skin.

Hormone Replacement Therapy Combats Ageing

During menopause, women usually develop an oestrogen deficiency, and doctors prescribe hormone replacement therapy to supplement oestrogen in the body. Especially women who have had a hysterectomy or stopped menstruating very early might need oestrogen.

Although hormone replacement therapy is in the first place not prescribed to improve skin and hair quality, the skin benefits greatly from it. It improves skin quality and hydration by stimulating collagen production in the dermis. Women on hormone replacement therapy often report a reduction in fine wrinkling. Unfortunately, deeper wrinkles don't show significant improvement. If the skin is not damaged by photoaging, it responds even better to hormone therapy.

Not all hormone replacement therapies are the same, though. Some contain high doses of oestrogen. Others have a combination of oestrogen and progesterone, which is particularly important for women who had a hysterectomy at a young age or experienced early menopause. Oestrogen alone stimulates growth in the uterus lining and poses a cancer risk.

Cancer Research U.K. is quite clear on the risk of hormone replacement therapy and cancer. There is some risk, but it is minimal. For some women, hormone replacement therapy's benefits outweigh the risks. Cancer Research U.K. recommends that women consult their doctors (Cancer Research UK, 2021).

Doctors consider a woman's personal and family medical history before prescribing hormone therapy. The following are taken into account: high blood pressure, thrombosis, stroke, heart disease, breast cancer, and gallbladder diseases.

Ageing is natural; premature ageing is not. Your skin is a barometer of what is going on inside your body. It shows when your hormones are acting up. Be aware of skin changes and see your doctor. Advances in science and skincare have made it possible to supplement your declining hormones and preserve skin quality for much longer without risking your health. You can have good skin quality at every age. Review the section at the end of this chapter for treatment options.

Inflammaging, the Secret Ageing Factor

There are two types of inflammation: acute and chronic inflammation:

- Acute inflammation usually occurs over a short period, and the affected area swells, becomes red, and feels warm. It can be treated and healed within a reasonable time and is not discussed here.

- Chronic inflammation happens gradually and often; you are not even aware of it. It can be caused by several factors such as exposure to chemicals, a foreign object, a seemingly unimportant injury, or repeated acute inflammation.

Inflammaging is a relatively new concept based on recent research. It means what the name says: accelerated ageing caused by low-grade chronic inflammation. It releases free radicals that contribute significantly to skin ageing.

Although silently and without you knowing, chronic low-grade inflammation damages your body and skin. Often, chronic inflammation is a symptom of another illness. Only when diagnosed with the primary disease will chronic inflammation come to the fore in many cases.

There's more to inflammation than meets the eye. It is a necessary process in the body and the immune system's natural response to injury. Inflammation is thus the body's way of healing itself.

Unfortunately, when inflammation continues indefinitely, it becomes a problem. Macrophages, white blood cells that help with immunity, may overproduce free radicals. Consequently, matrix-destroying enzymes break down the cell structure's proteins (collagen and elastin). The result is ageing skin, dryness, thinning, and wrinkles.

The overproduction of free radicals is called oxidation. Although life is not possible without oxygen, when oxidation goes unchecked, it can also destroy body tissue.

Chapter 3 on skincare ingredients discusses free radicals in more detail. In short, we are exposed to free radicals every day; therefore, chronic low-grade inflammation should be avoided as much as possible.

What can one do about chronic inflammation?

In ideal circumstances, antioxidants neutralise free radicals, and prevention is the best cure. Stimulating antioxidants in the body is the way to prevent oxidative stress. Oxidative stress happens when there is an imbalance between free radicals and antioxidants in the skin. There are not enough oxidants to counteract the damage done by free radicals. Oxidative stress plays a significant role in ageing, as it contributes to a reduction in collagen.

Healthy Living Prevents Chronic Inflammation

We hear it so often that the phrase 'a healthy lifestyle' has become a cliché.

- Excess weight adds oxidative stress to the organs. The best starting point is to maintain a healthy body weight.

- Eat a diet low in sugar and high in vegetables and fruits, whole grains, and lean proteins.

- Avoid all processed foods, as most are high in fats and sugars.

- Quit smoking – today. The effects of smoking on the skin are discussed in the next chapter.

- Manage your stress if you can't avoid it. Breathing exercises, mindfulness, meditation, and exercises such as walking and yoga are cheap and available. Do not under evaluate them because they are mostly free and readily available. And no, you are NOT too old for any of the above.

- Avoid pollution and harsh chemicals.

Medication for Chronic Inflammation

Over-the-counter medications are available. You can buy aspirin and ibuprofen at the pharmacy to reduce inflammation. However, they are not the answer over the long term, as they can cause other conditions. Experts linked the long-term use of aspirin and ibuprofen to kidney problems and peptic ulcer disease.

Speak to your doctor: Do not self-diagnose and self-treat indefinitely.

Your doctor might recommend corticosteroid shots. Corticosteroid is a type of hormone. It decreases inflammation effectively, but again, long-term use can be problematic. They can cause high blood pressure and osteoporosis.

Supplements containing vitamins A, C, and D, zinc (found in fish oil), and foods such as curcumin, ginger, garlic, cayenne, tomatoes, leafy greens like spinach and kale, and olive oil might help.

Quick Reminder

A well-kept woman does not strive to look younger but to be the best version of herself at every age.

Inflammaging is a hidden ageing factor. Chronic low-grade inflammation releases free radicals and destroys skin cells and structure.

Ageing is a natural process in the body and skin but is accelerated by external factors such as sun damage, pollution, and personal neglect.

Skin ageing happens in all layers of the face: epidermis, the membrane between epidermis and dermis, dermis, and the supporting fat layer at the bottom of the skin.

Menopause sees a decline in most hormones that regulate the production of skin proteins such as collagen and elastin.

Hormone replacement therapy is safe and contributes to many women's quality of life and improved skin.

Chapter 9:
Surgical and Non-Surgical Procedures to Combat Ageing

Everybody does what she needs. And if you want plastic surgery, and then feel better, why not? There is no law. I've nothing against using something to help your beauty – but do it in the good way, with intelligence.

It might be possible to divide the world into two groups: those who are pro-cosmetic procedures and those who oppose them.

Monica Bellucci, the Italian model and actress, who at 50-something was the oldest Bond girl ever, has some common-sense advice for women: If it makes you feel better, do it, but do it intelligently.

Surgical Procedures/Cosmetic Surgery

Cosmetic surgery developed from reconstructive surgery and is a relatively new development. Unfortunately, surgery is the only way to get rid of loose skin. Non-invasive procedures can treat wrinkles and age spots, but only surgery can remove excess skin permanently.

Where reconstructive surgery is done for medical reasons – correcting a congenital disability or injury – cosmetic surgery is done for aesthetic reasons. Some will go so far as to say it is pure vanity.

But public acceptance of cosmetic surgery has shifted over the last several years, and many more people are positive about it. Also, more women and men declare they would consider cosmetic surgery if possible.

Extensive media coverage has helped, bringing cosmetic surgery into our lounges and lives. Many celebrities now openly discuss their procedures. Furthermore, programmes such as *Nip/Tuck* and *Extreme Makeover* contributed to a growing acceptance of cosmetic surgery as a logical way to combat the signs of ageing. However, these programmes predominantly emphasise the positives of surgery – improved looks, self-acceptance, happiness, and a better social life (Rubin, 2018).

Despite the positives, cosmetic surgery also holds medical and emotional risks.

Emotional Impact and Medical Risks of Cosmetic Surgery

Cosmetic surgery, even when subtly done and well-executed, brings dramatic changes. More often than not, the change in appearance has emotional implications. It might be a good idea to ask yourself *why* you want to have the surgery. *What* are your expectations? *How* do you expect to look after the operation? *How* will your improved appearance change your life?

The decision to have plastic surgery is very personal. Your emotions might jump from excitement to guilt and even fear. Is it vain to spend so much money on appearance? Will friends and family judge you or, even worse, mock you? Only you can decide and see the process through despite others' opinions.

If you are deeply unhappy with your appearance, take the step but realise that getting rid of excess skin or the shape of your nose will not automatically make you happy. The best candidate for cosmetic surgery is probably already happy and grounded in a supportive family or circle of friends. But, being happy does not mean you can't strive to look or feel better. Happiness does not equal self-satisfaction but rather feeling good about yourself and continually striving to be kinder to yourself and others.

It might help to discuss it with friends and family, but a good starting point is to discuss it with the surgeon. Your surgeon will consider your medical history and ask questions about your general health, smoking, and weight fluctuations. Any surgery has risks, and the surgeon will not take a chance to operate on an unhealthy individual.

It is also vital to discuss your expectations; no surgeon can change you into Angelina Jolie. However, a cosmetic surgeon can remove the loose skin giving you a turkey neck or bags around the eyes. The surgeon will explain what you can and cannot expect. The human face is not perfectly symmetrical; consequently, when one aspect of the face is changed, the balance of the other features might also be affected.

It is important to speak about your expectations honestly. Don't feel rushed or anxious. You pay a lot of money and have the right to get answers to your questions. The better informed you are, the less nervous you will be. Ask your surgeon those nagging questions and listen to their advice.

Remember, having a facelift won't change your social life, get you more friends, or earn a raise at work. However, a facelift will give you the confidence to join a dating club, attend social meetings, and approach your boss about a promotion.

If you decide to have your turkey neck corrected or the excess skin around your eyes removed, focus on the future and be positive.

Surgery always has risks: It is a big decision. The following are not meant to scare you or put you off surgery, but you should know what can go wrong.

- Anaesthesia could have side effects such as pneumonia and blood clots.

- There may be wound infection, scarring, and bruising.

- There may be fluid build-up under the skin or wound complications.

- Unexpected bleeding might require a second operation.

- There may be numbness and tingling due to nerve damage.

Recovery and Downtime Can Be Long and Lonely

After the stress and trauma of surgery, the recovery period often proves to be equally traumatic. You will look terrible and might have pain. You will feel guilty and might even be depressed. You will check the mirror a thousand times a day and doubt you will recover.

Be prepared for the emotional ups and downs by having ready meals in the freezer, good books, and your favourite movies available. Once you can move freely, do those long-overdue tasks: tidying your underwear drawer or sorting your paperwork.

Keep your mind busy, and don't obsess over the bruising. Stay away from doctor google until you are well on the path to recovery. You don't need extra stress or to see problems where there are none.

Your wounds will heal as long as you follow the surgeon's instructions. Clean the wound as instructed, don't touch the area unnecessarily, and don't go into stress-eating mode.

The worst swelling and bruising will pass after two weeks, but actual healing can take months. Make sure you know what is expected and which symptoms might need a doctor's attention.

Red light therapy, discussed below, helps speed up recovery. On top of that, it is relaxing and can start about 24 hours after surgery or as soon as you can move without discomfort.

You will be rewarded for your patience when the bruising and swelling eventually subside and you can see the results. It is a magic moment when you know all the stress and hardship were worthwhile. Enjoy your improved appearance and be grateful.

Surgical Procedures

Facelift

Facial cosmetic surgery includes a full facelift (rhytidectomy) or several smaller procedures to improve a specific problematic area. Of course, a full facelift is an ultimate way to look younger, but it is expensive. Also, it is a big operation, and you will need at least a month's downtime.

In a traditional facelift, the surgeon makes small incisions around the ears and the hairline. The skin is separated from the underlying tissue, the muscles and other supporting tissues are tightened, and fat is removed from the neck. The surgeon then repositions the face's skin and removes excess skin. After recovery, barely visible scars run around the ear and hairline and can easily be covered by hair.

A deep-plane facelift involves lifting all the layers of the face, skin, fat, and muscles as a single unit.

Get a new hairstyle if you don't want people to know about your facelift. Everybody will think your new youthful appearance is because of the new cut and colour.

If you can't afford or stomach a traditional facelift, you can have a mini-facelift (on the lower face and neck). Or you might consider a mid-facelift (treating the cheek area) or a superficial musculoaponeurotic (SMAS) to lift the lower two-thirds of the face.

Different procedures will produce different outcomes, and discussing your worries and expectations with the surgeon is important. Tell your surgeon exactly what you want and listen to their advice.

Smaller Procedures

Consider a smaller procedure if you are generally happy with how you have aged but unhappy with drooping eyelids or a turkey neck. The surgeon often recommends non-invasive treatments such as botox or fillers to enhance the procedure's results.

Remove Excess Skin From the Eyelids

A blepharoplasty, removing excess skin around the eyes, is a popular and relatively small operation. It takes off years and is done on the lower, upper, or both eyelids. The light scar on the upper eyelid runs along the natural fold and is not visible. On the lower lid, it runs just below the lashes, entirely invisible after two or three weeks.

Fat Grafting

Your doctor can use your own fat to fill deep folds or smile lines from the nose to the mouth. Through liposuction, they get the fat from another part of your body, typically the abdomen or bottom. A special machine separates the fat from your blood and other fluids.

Fat grafting is a permanent type of filler for the deep nasal folds, lips, and hollow under-eyes. It is the answer to what doctors call volume loss; it can take years off and has little downtime.

You can go home on the same day but will have some bruising, swelling, and temporary numbness.

Ask Your Dentist for Botox

Yes, your dentist might have branched out into rejuvenating the lips and area around the mouth with a combination of botox and fillers. Dentists' knowledge of the area around the mouth and jaw makes them the ideal candidates to do botox and fillers to contour the lower half of the face.

One of the lesser known signs of ageing is a change in the upper lip. We are aware of the mouth corners turning down to give one a disgruntled look. However, the upper lip also becomes longer and thinner and loses its upward curve. Volume loss of soft tissue in the upper lip causes it to hang, and older women often have a long and unflattering look.

The mouth plays a vital role in expressing emotion, and a long upper lip adds to a tired appearance. More dentists now also inject the lips with dermal fillers and relax the muscles on both sides of the vertical groove between the nose and the upper lip. Your cupid's bow will curl upward ever so slightly and give you back a youthful expression.

Turkey Neck

There are several options to minimise a turkey neck, but cosmetic surgeons agree a neck lift is the best and only long-term solution. If surgery is not an option, discuss the following temporary solutions with your surgeon. Botox and laser treatments are discussed in more detail in the section 'Non-Surgical Procedures'.

- Thread lifting is a short procedure done under a local anaesthetic. The surgeon places fine threads just under the skin surface and lifts the neck. The threads stimulate collagen forming, but not all threads are the same. Research has proved that PLLA promotes collagen production for longer than PDO threads. PLLA threads also have tiny cones that attach to the tissue and increase volume. A thread lift lasts for about 18 months. Depending on the laxity of the skin and the amount of loose skin, different methods can be used: The crosshatch technique gives greater textural improvement and is recommended for people with a double chin. When there is still some laxity in the skin, the hammock technique effectively anchors the skin at the mastoid fascia. Linear threading is used in less severe cases of turkey neck.

- Ultherapy is a new non-invasive ultrasound treatment that delivers heat to the deeper layers of the skin and the neck muscles. It stimulates collagen forming, and the effect lasts for about two years.

- Botox relaxes those pertinent vertical muscles running down your neck. The effect lasts for about four months.

- Laser skin tightening is effective, especially if you don't have lots of loose skin. The results are not as good as surgery, and several sessions are usually necessary. Also, you will have to repeat this procedure regularly for maintenance.

Non-Surgical Procedures

Chapter 3 discusses skincare products and the key ingredients to hydrate and promote skin quality.

Non-surgical procedures have been discussed several times in this book. They predominantly aim to resurface and accelerate skin regeneration. They mostly remove or accelerate desquamation of the damaged epidermis and/or stimulate new cells to form.

Chemical Peels

A chemical peel removes the skin's top layers. Some chemical peels remove only the topmost layer, others go much deeper. It depends on the concentration of the chemical. Therefore, they are classified according to the lipo-hydroxy and trichloroacetic acid content and the pH. The longer the chemical stays on the face, the more effective it will be.

Unfortunately, chemical peels can be painful and might have severe side effects, like scarring and hyperpigmentation. Therefore, the dermatologist usually considers personal and family history of scarring and liver, kidney, and heart health. It is vital to choose a board-certified professional and follow their instructions to the T.

In particular, invasive chemical peels can cause infections. You might take antiviral medication before and after treatment to prevent infections. Furthermore, retinoids before treatment can help with healing. Staying out of the sun before and after chemical peels is vital, as the skin is extremely sensitive.

Superficial Peel

The weakest or most superficial chemical peel removes only the dead outer layer from the epidermis. Desquamation is accelerated, and natural enzymes stimulate further exfoliation of dead cells. It helps with acne, fine wrinkles, and uneven skin tone. It can be repeated every few weeks. The discomfort during the procedure is moderate, but you will have a small hand-held fan to cool down the stinging.

Medium Peel

The medium-depth peels remove dead cells from the epidermis and go deeper to the upper layer of the dermis. Repeated medium peels treat acne scars and uneven skin tone. Some women find the discomfort level high and ask for a topical numbing agent.

You may use over-the-counter pain medication and ice packs. Do not pick the crust, and allow yourself at least 14 days to heal.

Deep Peel

A deep peel is seriously invasive and must be done under controlled hygienic conditions by a certified medical practitioner.

Deep peels go into the reticular dermis. Although highly uncomfortable, the deep peel reduces deep wrinkles, scars, and precancerous growths. The results are usually very satisfying. The epidermis is more structurally balanced, and melanocytes are distributed evenly. Furthermore, it also restores and distributes melanin evenly in the basal cells. The basal layer membrane becomes thicker. New collagen and elastin are formed.

Your doctor will probably give you a sedative, apply a numbing cream, and you will get fluids intravenously. Your doctor will cover your skin in a surgical dressing, and you must soak and apply ointment for about 14 days.

You can go home after the treatment but are not allowed to drive. Chemical peels cause swollen, red, and irritated skin. The deeper the peel, the more the skin will be affected. Prepare yourself for a few weeks' downtime – physically and emotionally.

At some stage, you will wonder whether it was worthwhile at all. Don't despair; you will see the results after a few weeks. Although your skin will be red for a long time, you can cover the redness with foundation as soon as your doctor gives the go-ahead.

Visible Light Devices

LED Light Therapy

Light therapy is a non-invasive treatment with little or no downtime, with excellent results for acne, inflammation, fine lines, and wound healing. It uses different wavelengths of light to activate regeneration processes in the skin.

The lights do not contain any UV radiation; consequently, they hold no risk of cancer. The good news is that LED light therapy is now available as a home treatment. Previously, only salons offered light therapy, which was costly. However, hand-held products do not come cheap.

Red light therapy is primarily used for treating the epidermis. Cells in the epidermis absorb the light, and this causes collagen production. Simultaneously, it reduces inflammation and improves blood flow. Because red light therapy is healing, it is often used after invasive procedures such as micro-needling.

Blue light therapy goes deeper and targets the sebaceous glands at the bottom of the hair follicles. The blue light reduces sebum production and prevents acne breakouts.

Red and blue lights are often combined for even better results. Yellow light therapy supposedly penetrates deeper than red light and helps with removing fine lines. Green light therapy again claims to heal those tiny broken capillaries. However, more research on the benefits of yellow and green light therapy is necessary.

Salon treatments are more potent with better results. You will have to go for several sessions to see a significant improvement in skin quality, though. Remember that you can't get light therapy while on Accutane treatment.

Furthermore, repeated maintenance sessions are necessary because natural cell turnover reduces collagen production. Therefore, consider investing in a good home product. It is essential to follow the instructions. Side effects are minimal, but take special care around the eyes. Some users experience redness, swelling, and dryness.

There are many versions available. Choose one that suits your pocket, but remember: It will only work if you use it regularly.

Ablative and Nonablative Laser

Laser resurfacing improves age spots, wrinkles, sun damage, mild scars, and skin texture. People with UV photodamage might benefit from laser therapy. Especially people with dark skin are at a higher risk for hyperpigmentation and scarring during laser treatment. Consult a dermatologist and follow their advice.

Unfortunately, laser therapy does not improve a turkey neck and does not improve sagging of excessive skin.

Non-ablative resurfacing stimulates collagen production. As it is less invasive, several sessions are usually necessary. The results are not as dramatic as ablative therapy, but there is no downtime.

Ablative resurfacing is more invasive and painful, with 14 days to one month of downtime. It is not a decision you can make on the spur of the moment. Think it through properly after speaking to a dermatologist. Healing takes longer and can be emotionally exhausting.

Your doctor will check your medical history, current medication, pregnancy, other conditions, and previous treatments. You will have a thorough physical examination also. You should ask about the treatment process and discuss your expectations about the results.

Sometimes, you will have to take precautionary medication to prevent viral infections. It is an outpatient procedure, but you will get sedation and a numbing cream on the treated area.

During the procedure, an intense light beam destroys the epidermis and heats the cells in the dermis. The heat stimulates collagen production, which improves skin texture and tone. It is quite a lengthy process, and treating the whole face can take up to two hours.

The real challenge comes afterward. Your face will be raw, swollen, and itchy. Your doctor will probably wrap your face in a watertight dressing. You might need pain medication and ice packs. Prepare ahead for two to four weeks of staying out of the sun.

The recovery time is usually difficult, as you look terrible and seldom want to let other people see you with a red, scabby face.

Keep busy with a good book, special magazines, and uplifting TV programs. Keep positive and remind yourself that the results will be worthwhile for years.

If you decide to go the laser way, you will have to commit to wearing sunscreen every day, summer and winter, forever.

Radiofrequency (RF)

Radiofrequency is used for skin tightening and can repair sun damage also.

It sends energy waves into the skin that stimulates collagen production. It is a non-surgical way to tighten the skin. Laser and light therapy use light to heat the skin into collagen production, whereas radiofrequency uses energy.

Radiofrequency uses energy in electromagnetic waves like your microwave and x-rays do. However, skincare energy waves are one billion times weaker (Yetman, 2020).

The procedure is painless and takes about an hour. During radiofrequency therapy, the device maintains a temperature of 46°C (115°F) on the skin for three minutes. The body reacts by releasing heat-shock proteins that cause collagen production (Yetman, 2020).

Radiofrequency treatment is rated safe, with temporary redness and swelling being the most likely side effects. However, people with darker skin should be careful, as hyperpigmentation and scarring can occur. If you are prone to pigmentation or scarring, speak to a dermatologist before having the treatment done.

Microneedling

Microneedles prick the skin with tiny needles and cause minute little wounds. Your body wants to heal the wounds and sends collagen and elastin to the area.

It helps improve acne, alopecia (hair loss), enlarged pores, hyperpigmentation, sun damage, fine lines, and reduced elasticity. The good news is that women with dark skin can have microneedling, as the risk for spots and scarring is limited.

A dermatologist or certified beautician can do microneedling, and hand-held home devices are also available. The home device will not give the same effect, though, as the needles do not go as deep. Because it causes wounds (although minute), hygiene and sterilised equipment are vital; check the credentials and certification of the professional carefully.

As with other invasive treatments, your skin will be numbed with a cream. The skin could be red and slightly painful depending on how deep the needles pierce. Bruising and bleeding are rare. The risk of infection is low if done in sterile conditions.

Microneedling is much cheaper than laser treatment and less invasive, but several sessions are necessary.

Cryolipolysis

Cryolipolysis is a fat-freezing technology that kills fat and allows the body to get rid of dead fat cells naturally. It all began with researchers studying the effect of frostbite on fat. They found that fat freezes at a much higher temperature than the skin and developed a device that freezes the fat: Two paddles hold the targeted area for an extended period to freeze and kill the fat cells. As the body's immune system gets rid of the dead fat tissue, the results are not immediately visible. It is suitable for those problematic areas, such as saddlebags on the hips.

All surgical procedures might have side effects. Speaking to your doctor about all procedures and risks is vital.

Dermal Fillers

The beauty of fillers is that one sees immediate results. You walk in with deep nasal folds, and 15 minutes later, you walk out with flattened-out folds. You might be slightly sore and have tiny prick marks, but nothing that a good foundation can't cover.

Soft-tissue or dermal fillers give structure and volume to the face, especially around the nose and mouth. It is the solution for drooping mouth corners. It is also used to even out scar tissue, erase fine lines, and rejuvenate the hands.

There are many fillers on the market. They all contain a combination of the following: collagen, hyaluronic acid, calcium hydroxylapatite, and poly-L-lactic acid.

Unfortunately, fillers are only temporary and depend on the precise cocktail used. Collagen, for example, depletes sooner than hyaluronic acid. Poly-L-lactic acid can last up to three years.

Dermal fillers have slight side effects, including redness, swelling, and bruising. It usually improves within days and can be covered by make-up.

Warning: It is relatively easy to have fillers done, and the procedure takes about 15 minutes. Because injecting fillers seems an uncomplicated process, many unqualified people offer filler treatment at home or at parties. Even if the hygiene is impeccable, in untrained hands, you could end up looking unnatural and unsymmetrical. Spend more; wait until you can get an appointment and have it done professionally.

Platelet-Rich Plasma (PRP)

The chapter on hyperpigmentation discusses platelet-rich fillers, which minimise hyperpigmentation. It is also a dermal filler to remove fine lines, give volume, and diminish scars.

To recap: The procedure is done by a dermatologist who separates a patient's blood sample in a centrifuge machine. The patient is injected with plasma sourced from their own blood. The plasma is rich in growth factors that stimulate collagen production. One benefit is that it is unlikely that you will be allergic to your own plasma. The effect lasts between six and nine months.

You will receive a numbing cream and some form of sedative before treatment. The treatment takes about an hour and has minimal side effects. You will receive a list of instructions to follow. No make-up is allowed for three days at least.

In contrast to other dermal fillers, platelet-rich plasma fillers do not have the immediate 'wow' factor. However, skin texture improves gradually over the following weeks. The full effect will only be visible about three months after treatment. Dermatologists recommend repeat treatments after six to eight weeks.

Botulinum Toxin (Botox)

(Botox is a registered trademark but has become a collective term for all types of botulinum injections. It is used as a collective term here.)

Everybody jokes about botox, but millions of men and women use it successfully. Different areas of the face improve with botox injections: frown lines between the brows, crow's feet, horizontal lines on the forehead, lines at the mouth corners, and uneven texture on the chin.

Botox has a bad name, partly because of the grotesque images of celebrities who supposedly overdo botox and partly because it is derived from a known toxin. However, botox in minute quantities has been safely used for medical and cosmetic purposes for many decades.

Medical treatment with botox helps with eye spasms, excessive sweating, migraine, and some bladder disorders.

But we are interested in how botox can help counteract the visible signs of ageing.

Botox is naturally present in nature – the soil, water, forests, and even in the intestines of some animals and fish. In nature, it is not problematic unless the spores multiply and the cell population increases to form a neurotoxin responsible for botulism, a kind of food poisoning.

The botox used in cosmetic treatments is safe and authorised by national health organisations. It temporarily paralyses the muscles and relaxes wrinkles and lines.

As with all cosmetic procedures, only a qualified person should do botox. Botox in the wrong hands could make you the neighbourhood's resident joke.

Quick Reminder

There is help to age well: Surgical and non-surgical procedures can do wonders to combat the signs of ageing.

Surgery is a big decision; it is costly and causes immense emotions before and after surgery.

All surgeries carry risks; ensure you are informed before making a decision.

Recovery from surgery takes time. Swelling and bruising heal in about 14 days, but internal healing might take months.

Non-surgical procedures are excellent for acne and less severe signs of ageing, such as fine wrinkles, inflammation, hyperpigmentation, and dry skin.

Chemical peels are suitable for most signs of ageing but can be very uncomfortable. The lighter the peel, the less the pain level. Deep peels take much longer to heal, but the results are much better than lighter peels.

Light therapy has little downtime and helps with fine lines, inflammation, and wound healing. It has to be repeated several times, though.

Laser therapy improves all ageing symptoms, but people with dark skin risk hyperpigmentation. Non-ablative laser therapy has no actual downtime but must be repeated over a period of time for visible results.

Ablative laser therapy is much more invasive, and downtime is at least 14 days. The results are very good.

Radiofrequency helps with skin-tightening and requires minimal downtime.

Microneedling helps with hair loss, hyperpigmentation, sun damage, and fine lines. Several treatments are necessary.

Platelet-rich plasma injections from the patient's blood are a dermal filler with virtually no risk of allergies. However, it takes longer to show results.

Fat grafting is also a type of derma filler. Fat from the patient is prepared and injected. It is usually a day procedure, and some bruising is possible.

Botox for frown lines, crow's feet, and a fresher appearance is not toxic, as millions of men and women can testify.

Chapter 10:
Are You Destroying Your Own Beauty?

Genetics loads the gun; the environment pulls the trigger.

Your genes determine skin colour, natural moisture level, and tendency to develop wrinkles or acne. But there, your genetics stops: Your behaviour and how you care for yourself and your skin are more important for skin quality than genetics. You cannot change the colour of your skin, but you can protect yourself from sun damage. You cannot change dry skin to oily, but you can moisturise your skin.

Treating your skin and body well contributes more to your skin health than your genes. You might have inherited perfect skin from your mother; how you treat it will determine your skin quality. Not the best genes in the world can protect the skin against UV radiation, smoking, and an unhealthy lifestyle.

Genetics loads the gun, and you and the environment pull the trigger.

Behaviour and Environmental Ageing Factors

The previous chapters discuss natural ageing and the processes in the skin that slow cell regeneration and deplete the skin's natural moisture levels. Genes and the passing of years are not the only factors in skin ageing. Diet, exercise, lifestyle, and the environment may override good genes and damage the skin extensively.

In this chapter, you will learn about these environmental factors and personal habits that could wreak havoc on your skin.

Experts agree that UV radiation is the single most dangerous factor contributing to skin cancer and damaged skin. This book does not discuss skin cancer, as it is a severe medical issue; only doctors should deal with it. However, the fact that UV radiation plays a major role in malignant skin growths illustrates how important protection against sunburn is.

UV Radiation: The Skin's Worst Enemy

Why is UV radiation so dangerous? What happens in the skin that causes so much damage?

Chapter 5 on hyperpigmentation discusses the UV radiation's different wavelengths and their detrimental effect on different layers of the skin. UVA, UVB, and UVC damage the skin in their own way. Their damage is called photoaging.

Photoaging

Long-term exposure to UV radiation causes skin wrinkles, sagging skin, roughness, yellowish skin tone, small burst capillaries, and hyperpigmentation. In short, UV radiation ages skin prematurely and affects nearly every cell and natural substance in the skin. Experts use the term photoaging to describe the multiple ways in which UV radiation damages the skin:

- Collagen formation is reduced; therefore, the matrix (the connective tissue mainly consisting of collagen and elastin that gives structure to and supports the skin).

- The fibroblasts in the dermis are damaged, reducing collagen and elastin production.

- Excess sugars accumulate in the skin, interfering with the forming of the skin's proteins, collagen, and elastin.

- Natural hyaluronic acid production, the natural lubricator in the skin, is reduced.

- The keratinocytes in the epidermis are destroyed, causing DNA damage.

- DNA damage results in inflammation, cell death, and in severe cases, skin cancer.

- The release of free radicals leads to oxidative stress, with devastating results for skin cells.

- Photoaging inhibits the enzymes that induce antioxidants; consequently, natural antioxidants cannot be formed to neutralise the free radicals.

- Damaged cells lead to fat oxidation that breaks down the fatty acids in the skin. Fatty acids provide the energy necessary for new cells to form.

- Free radicals shorten the telomeres that protect the chromosomes. Chromosomes are necessary for the long-term survival of the cell.

Smoking

Smoking also severely damages the skin. Tobacco smoking is a global health problem. It contributes to cancer, coronary heart disease, stroke, damaged blood vessels, and lung diseases.

One can often identify a smoker by just looking at their skin: The stratum corneum is thick and dry with an uneven skin tone. The upper lip is darker with numerous vertical lines. Also, the eyes show squinting lines with under-eye bags.

Unfortunately, mouth hygiene suffers from smoking, and gum disease causes bad breath. Yellow teeth and fingers, sagging skin, even cataracts – the list gets longer and longer. Also, the longer you smoke, the more your skin and appearance will deteriorate.

Smoking slows wound healing and alleviates several skin diseases, such as acne and hair loss.

Nicotine narrows the blood vessels; consequently, less oxygen reaches the cells. Smoking causes a chemical reaction in the skin, damaging the proteins in the matrix, collagen, and elastin. It further causes oxidative stress, allowing free radicals to damage skin cells.

The good news is that some damage can be reversed when you quit smoking. The information in this guide will help you understand your skin and look after it better, and within weeks you will notice improvement.

Pollution

The skin barrier has been mentioned several times in this book, indicating how important this outermost layer of the skin is. Among other things, the skin barrier protects the skin from pollution. Pollution accelerates ageing and skin conditions such as acne, eczema, and psoriasis.

When the skin barrier is thin and weak, pollutants can penetrate and deplete the skin's natural lipids. These pollutants also damage collagen production and the skin's DNA.

Air pollution

Air pollution is known as particulate matter (PM), or harmful chemicals. The ozone suffers from industrial operations: soot, paints, varnishes, fuels storage, factory emissions, construction, power plants, mines, refuse incinerators, and exhaust fumes from road, rail, and air traffic. Occurrences such as volcanic activities and forest fires also release pollutants.

Women living in highly polluted areas have to take special care. Although smog particles are mostly too big to penetrate the skin barrier, the health risks are significant.

To prevent premature ageing and skin damage, moisturise regularly and always wear sunscreen during the day. Also, do not over-exfoliate, as this might further thin the skin barrier. Topical antioxidants containing vitamin C and E help counteract the free radicals released by pollution.

Make-up Damage

Many women can't bear facing the world without make-up. Some even feel naked without foundation, blusher, and a touch of lipstick. There is nothing wrong with make-up per se: It's a woman's best friend on those days when things don't go your way. Wearing make-up when you feel low lifts self-esteem and gives you the energy to tackle life's challenges.

However, you have to use the correct make-up for your skin type. Ensure that your foundation does not dry your skin or makes it too oily. Does it contain ingredients that could contribute to your skin sensitivity? Keep a list of sudden skin reactions when you use any new product. You might find that you have an allergic reaction to a specific chemical.

Also, check the ingredients, especially for parabens (harmful preservatives), discussed in Chapter 3.

Harsh ingredients can weaken the skin barrier, allowing dirt and pathogens to enter the pores. And yes, your mother was right when she said never to sleep with make-up. Make-up combines with surface dirt particles and clogs your pores. It is even worse if you don't apply sunscreen: UV radiation causes ageing, and its effect is worsened by old make-up.

Furthermore, sleeping with make-up allows surface free radicals to damage cells and weaken the barrier.

Do not work out with make-up, as the oil glands open during exercise and make-up will penetrate the pores, clogging them. This contributes to acne, inflammation, and fine lines.

Check the make-up's expiry date as it might no longer be effective and, even worse, might contain harmful bacteria. It goes without saying: Never share make-up and expose your skin to someone else's germs.

Your skin barrier protects you. Return the favour and protect your skin barrier by diligently applying moisturisers and sunscreen.

Alcohol and the Skin

Global statistics about alcohol abuse are scary: It plays a role in more than 200 diseases. It contributes to 5,1% of global medical expenditure. Approximately 13,5% of global deaths are alcohol-related. Alcohol contributes to many behavioural and mental disorders and causes significant social, emotional, and economic distress (WHO Fact Sheet, 2022).

Signs of Alcohol and Ageing

Heavy social drinking does not necessarily mean someone is an alcoholic, but excess alcohol consumption, unfortunately, leaves tell-tale signs on the skin:

- A yellowish tint and dry skin are often the first signs of heavy drinking. Alcohol dehydrates the skin, and dry skin accelerates ageing.

- Heavy drinkers are often recognised by the red spiderweb patches of broken fine capillaries on the cheeks.

- Fat and volume loss in the mid-face give a heavy drinker a hollow appearance.

- A heavy drinker's eyes age much quicker, and a grey ring forms around the corneas. Where this ring is usually found in people 80 years or older, heavy drinkers develop it decades earlier.

What Does Alcohol Abuse Do to the Skin?

Heavy drinkers have a vitamin deficiency and chronic inflammation, which prevent the skin from regenerating itself. Also, persistent inflammation causes broken capillaries and redness in the face.

Alcohol dehydrates the body. It is a diuretic; in other words, you go to the bathroom frequently. The body loses the electrolytes necessary to keep body fluids balanced through urination. Crude as it might sound, you flush your health down the toilet by drinking too much.

Your body naturally produces vasopressin, a hormone that retains water and keeps your body and skin hydrated. Alcohol reduces vasopressin production, and you urinate more frequently.

Alcohol also causes oxidative stress, releases free radicals that destroy collagen, and age the skin prematurely. One usually thinks alcohol helps one fall asleep, but heavy drinking causes disturbed sleep. Drunken sleep does not refresh but taps the body of energy, accelerating ageing in the skin, body, and psyche.

Worst Alcohol Types for the Skin

Although any amount of excessive alcohol is harmful to your skin, certain types of alcohol damage the skin more severely.

Dark alcohol such as *whiskey and brandy are particularly bad* for the skin. They contain congeners and some chemicals that worsen hangovers. A hangover dehydrates the skin and leaves it dry and dull. Brandy has low levels of methanol, which further dries the skin and can contribute to eczema and dermatitis. Please note that minute quantities of methanol, such as a single brandy, are not toxic. (Illegally produced alcohol can be deadly because of high methanol content.)

Cocktails, the favourites of many women, contain lots of sugar. Excessive sugar in the skin triggers the hormone IGF-1, leading to oil overproduction and causing acne. Sugars also cause inflammation and worsen glycation. Glycation in the skin occurs when the sugar molecules attach themselves to collagen proteins and break them down. Margarita might be the worst of the cocktails, as it contains sugar and salt.

Red wine contains antioxidants; consequently it is mistakenly lauded for being healthy. However, red wine is often unfiltered, making it harder for the kidneys and liver. Red wine causes flushing and blotchy skin because it opens the blood vessels in the skin. It also releases histamine, which further contributes to redness.

White wine is also high in sugar, and too many glasses will have the same effect as cocktails. Sugar causes inflammation, and persistent inflammation will damage the cells. Overdoing white wine will make your skin dull and rough.

Beer in limited amounts is slightly less damaging because it contains antioxidants. It is not a ticket to drink excessively; beer does not have an abundance of antioxidants.

Lighter coloured drinks such as *vodka, gin, white rum, and sake* have fewer additives and sugars. They are processed quicker, and thus your body gets rid of them quicker. They are not too bad for the skin in limited quantities, but too much will harm you and your skin in the long term.

Tequila has less sugar; thus, it is better processed by the body. Have a small tequila without the salt and stick to soda water for the rest of the night.

Non-alcoholic alternatives are growing in popularity, and many alcohol-free mocktails, beers, and wines are on the market. However, do not have them without studying the labels and checking the sugar content. Too many sugars are very bad for the skin and weight.

A good idea is to alternate your drinks with water and soda water. It will help you cut your alcohol consumption dramatically and do your skin and body a favour.

Foods Bad for the Skin

High-Fat Diet

Everything one eats eventually affects the skin as the biggest organ in the body. The dangers of high-fat diets are well documented: It is a significant contributor to obesity, diabetes, fatty liver, and coronary heart diseases. Too high fat levels also affect the skin severely, as it impacts the fat tissue and the lipid composition in the skin.

Not all fats are bad: The body needs fats to function optimally, and healthy amounts of fat should be included in the diet. Use only limited quantities of the following *oils for cooking*: avocado, canola, fish, cottonseed, flax, linseed, margarine, palm, peanut, safflower, sesame, and soybean. Please note that avocados, fish, and many of the above are healthy; their oils are less beneficial.

What Do Too High Fats Do to the Skin?

Bad fats (polyunsaturated fats) are liquid at room temperature and solid when cooled. They are unstable when exposed to oxygen, light, or heat. Also, they do not contain hydrogen atoms that protect skin cells against free radicals. When eaten, these fats have already been chemically changed and cause oxidative stress.

This means that high amounts of fat release uncontrolled numbers of free radicals that cause inflammation. Inflammation destroys the skin's proteins, collagen, and elastin. It affects the skin's natural support and structure, the matrix. Chronic low-grade inflammation also causes age spots and pigmentation.

Also, large amounts of unhealthy fat affect thyroid function. The thyroid is vital for general health, as it determines one's metabolism and the rate energy is used. A lazy thyroid causes, among other things, weight gain and fatigue. The skin also suffers from poor blood circulation, toxin accumulation, and a dull complexion.

Furthermore, the digestive system struggles to digest high-fat content. Slow digestion impacts the secretion of enzymes that help with protein formation in the skin. It also makes the skin more prone to parasite infection and inflammation.

Sugar

Sugar is sweet, but its sweetness is short-lived. It does not only contribute to weight gain and many associated diseases but also bad skin quality.

The chapter on acne highlights how excess sugar intake causes glycation and contributes to breakouts. In addition, sugar also causes several other skin problems.

What Do Excess Sugars Do to the Skin?

Let's catch up quickly on glycation and acne's relation to sugar. Sugar is an inflammatory food. It triggers inflammation in the skin. It can also increase sebum production, making the skin more prone to acne. Despite higher sebum production, the skin will age quicker.

Glycation occurs naturally in the bloodstream when insulin cannot handle the high level of sugars. The sugar molecules look for another destination and attach themselves to the proteins in the skin – collagen and elastin. They break down, and the skin structure is damaged.

Avoid Hidden Sources of Sugar

People think of sugar only in its obvious form, like added sugar to drinks or dishes, but there are many hidden forms of sugar. Most carbohydrates – bread, pasta, rice, pastries – convert into sugar. So-called healthy foods – honey and fruit juice – have high sugar content.

Chemically Processed Foods

Chemically processed foods usually have lots of fats and sugars. In addition, chemically processed foods also contain trans fats, which are very bad for health. Trans fats are not natural but chemically manufactured by adding hydrogen to liquid vegetable fats. It results in a solid consistency, easier to add flavour, and a longer shelf life, thus making it more economical.

Health experts warn against trans fats; consequently, most countries have banned them. Still, many foods do contain some trans fats. Be careful when buying processed foods and check the ingredient list for 'partially hydrogenated oil'.

You might inadvertently create trans fats when frying food in margarine or certain vegetable oils. Every time such oils are reheated, more trans fats are formed. Be careful of food outlets that might reuse old oils. A diet of chemically processed foods is undeniably bad for skin health.

What Do Trans Fats Do to the Skin?

Trans fats block the arteries and thus cause inflammation. As we have learnt from previous chapters, inflammation triggers a series of chemical processes involving the release of free radicals, skin protein breakdown, skin structure damage, and sun damage.

Down the line, trans fats make the skin more vulnerable to UV radiation and photoaging. They contribute to dehydration, wrinkling, rough texture, and a thinning epidermis.

Your body will initially react negatively when you stop eating processed foods. You might experience headaches and irritability – signs that your body has become used to ill-treatment. After a few days, you will see an improvement in skin texture, and your skin quality will improve significantly with consistent avoidance of chemically processed foods.

Nutrients That Benefit the Skin

Healthy skin needs several natural nutrients for the natural biological processes to occur. Good nutrients not only keep the skin healthy but can also repair damaged cells in the skin and other organs. Eating healthily is essential for skin health and anti-ageing.

Water

Water is vital, and without water, your skin will be dehydrated. Check for a simple hydration test in the chapter on ageing. None of the normal body or skin processes is possible without water. It is a solvent that carries nutrients and waste, gives volume, and regulates body temperature.

A lack of proper hydration will age the skin. However, it is not true that water eliminates wrinkles and shrinks pores. Nonetheless, it's necessary to drink at least 2,5 litres of water every day for the skin to function properly (Raymond, 2021).

The good news is that you may count sugar-free drinks and your favourite cuppa when tallying the prescribed amount of daily water.

Trace Elements

Trace elements are those minute amounts of minerals found in the body. One might think they are insignificant, but your body needs them, and so does your skin. They contribute to skin immunity and the fight against inflammation.

Copper helps with the forming of fibroblasts in the dermis. It helps strengthen the matrix by cross-linking the collagen and elastin fibres. It improves skin elasticity and stimulates an antioxidant enzyme with anti-inflammatory properties. It also plays a role in melanin production, responsible for skin and hair colour.

Zinc is prevalent in the epidermis and helps to keep the keratinocytes healthy. In the dermis, it helps with collagen and elastin production. In addition, zinc is also an excellent anti-inflammatory, fights free radicals, and helps in wound healing. Its ability to produce enzymes that fight inflammation also helps against acne.

Zinc is a stalwart in sunscreen as it protects against UV radiation by reflecting the rays.

It is well-known that *iron* plays a significant role in haemoglobin and in carrying oxygen from the lungs to the various body parts. A shortage of iron can cause the skin to lighten because the red blood cells shrink.

However, iron also plays a role in hair and nail growth. It also assists in the healing of wounds and bruising.

Vitamins in Diet

Chapter 3 discusses the role of vitamins in skincare products. It is not enough to apply vitamins; one should buy fresh fruits and vegetables for vitamins. Vitamins provide antioxidants, the body's warriors against free radicals.

Although antioxidants are taken in through food, they are not nutrients but chemical properties. They stop damage to skin cells by stabilising the unbalanced electrons in free radicals.

- Vitamin D: Salmon, tuna, and cod have natural vitamin D, and many cereals are also fortified by added vitamin D. The sun plays a role in vitamin D absorption. Spending about ten minutes in the sun every day is sufficient. The body effectively absorbs vitamin D supplements. Vitamin D is important for healthy cells and even skin tone.

- Vitamin B: The leafy green vegetables contain most of the eight vitamin Bs. Salmon, eggs, oysters, and legumes also are sources of vitamin Bs. Vitamin Bs are instrumental in changing carbohydrates and proteins into energy, thus preventing fat build-up in the skin. They fight inflammation and prevent pigmentation.

- Vitamin C: Citrus fruits, strawberries, and leafy green vegetables – the healthy stuff – will provide natural vitamin C. It is a potent antioxidant and helps the skin in several ways.

- Vitamin E: Nuts and seeds have vitamin E and are also available in an oral supplement. Vitamin E is also an antioxidant and fights inflammation. It prevents dryness because it balances the sebum production.

- Vitamin K: Leafy green vegetables provide vitamin K. It helps against blood clotting and wound healing. Vitamin K is good for stretch marks, tiny broken capillaries, scars, and pigmentation.

Proteins

The skin's primary proteins, collagen and elastin, are discussed in every chapter of this book. They are the backbone of the skin in many ways: they provide structure, repair tissues, supply energy, and are instrumental in skin renewal.

A diet of healthy animal and plant proteins is essential for healthy skin. Not all proteins are necessarily healthy, though. Avoid those with high fat and salt content. Fish and plant proteins usually contain most of the amino acids necessary to provide energy for skin cell regulation.

Proteins fight inflammation, provide antioxidants, and generally make the skin stronger and healthier.

Foods such as salmon, eggs, Greek yoghurt, nuts, and seeds are obvious choices. You might also try fermented foods like tofu. Tofu contains isoflavones that, according to studies, improve skin quality in ageing skin (USSEC, 2016).

Omega Fatty Acids

Omega-3 fatty acids are a vital part of the skin's natural lipids to maintain volume. Volume loss, unfortunately, goes with ageing. It is partly caused by redistributing the subcutaneous fat layer at the bottom of the skin. However, the lipids in the other skin layers also form part of the skin structure and prevent you from looking hollow and sunken. A healthy diet and regular moisturising replenish skin lipids.

There are three types of Omega-3 fatty acids, and each plays a different role in the skin. ALA provides energy for cell function. DHA keeps cell membranes soft and moist, and thus helps prevent wrinkles.

EPA helps with oil management and keeps the skin moisturised. If you have wondered about those little red bumps on the upper arms, those are damaged keratinocytes in the hair follicles, and EPA helps to prevent them. Sufficient EPA in the skin also prevents acne. In general, Omega-3 fatty acids help against skin ageing.

Omega-6 plays a vital role in hair health. Thus, eating soybean, corn, nuts, and seeds will improve hair loss and texture.

Furthermore, Omega-6 helps with moisturising and wound healing. It is vital for preventing skin irritations, acne, and hyperpigmentation.

Include the following substances and nutrients in your daily diet to prevent skin ageing: water, trace elements, vitamins, proteins, and fatty acids.

Exercise for a Healthy Skin

Exercise increases heart rate and blood flow, and its benefits for general and heart health are well-known. Increased blood circulation in the skin contributes significantly to its health. Fresh blood brings oxygen and nutrients to the cells, enabling them to regenerate optimally. Once the blood has delivered the good stuff, it takes away the waste, toxins, and free radicals to the liver, where they are detoxified.

Exercise also releases stress that lessens the secretion of stress hormones. Cortisol stimulates sebum production that clogs pores and causes acne. Exercise can thus help fight acne caused by stress.

However, you must manage UV radiation during outdoor exercise. Never exercise in the middle of the day when the sun is at its hottest and most dangerous. The best protection against sunburn is sunscreen. Wear sunscreen even during early morning or later afternoon exercise sessions.

Women with acne are often worried about the effect of sweat. You can still work out, but don't wear make-up during exercise. Make-up and sweat can clog the pores. A light moisturiser and sunscreen keep the skin soft and the damaging rays at bay.

Shower or clean the skin gently immediately after a workout. It is essential to remove the sweat, bacteria, and oils that can clog the pores.

Quick Reminder

Genetics loads the gun, and the environment (and you) pull the trigger.

You can control your exposure to UV radiation and the devastating effects of photoaging.

Smoking ages your skin, and only you can stop nicotine from destroying your appearance.

Alcohol abuse ages your skin, and only you can stop drinking too much.

A high-fat diet causes skin a variety of problems and causes chronic inflammation. You have to choose to eat less fatty food.

Sugar triggers inflammation and destroys skin health; only you can choose healthier snacks.

Processed foods contain too high amounts of sugar and fats. In addition, processed foods contain trans fat – banned in most countries but still on our plates nearly every day.

Exercise increases blood flow and brings fresh oxygen and nutrients to the skin.

You cannot control the many forms of environmental pollution, but you can protect your skin barrier from absorbing harmful chemicals.

Chapter 11:
Tattoo Regret

My body is my journal, and my tattoos are my story.

People get tattoos for many reasons, like telling their individual stories or reflecting their loyalties. However, all tattoos have one thing in common: They are difficult to remove.

Johnny Depp's right arm depicts his first tattoo, a Native American in profile wearing a feathered headdress. He got inked to honour his great-grandmother, who was Cherokee, something he's very proud of. Many tattoos later, the actor seems happy with his life story told on his skin. Tattoos as body art date back thousands of years; archaeologists found that the Egyptians tattooed enslaved people to mark them.

But tattoos were not only for slaves; through the years, people from all walks of life decorated themselves with tattoos.

In the early 1800s, Jermyn Street in London was the centre of high society and had a tattoo salon (Michalak, 2022). Legend has it that Winston Churchill and his mother, the flamboyant Jennie Spencer-Churchill (later Porch and still later Cornwallis-West), had tattoos, but historians doubt that it is true (Rove, 2021). Still, the fact that these colourful public personalities could have tattoos seems to interest people even today. It shows that tattoos are potent symbols of defiance, adventure, and mystique.

Why Do People Get Tattoos?

The reasons for getting tattoos vary, but one thing applies to all tattoos: They are complicated to remove. Psychologists declare people get tattoos for the following reasons:

- Some tattoos are cultural markers. For example, a tattoo signifies clan and tribe in the Maori tradition. Tattoos often mark gang and prison syndicate members, but many modern social groups such as bikers or rock bands have tattoos. And they are good citizens with no criminal connections. To them, their distinctive tattoos are a symbol of belonging and exclusivity.

- Many people get tattoos to honour an intensely personal and meaningful event. In 1988, Johnny Depp had a heart tattooed on his left arm that reads 'Betty Sue', his mother's name. She passed away many years later, on May 20 2016, after a protracted illness. A young father might get a tattoo to mark the birth of a child, or a madly in love couple tattoo their partner's name in a heart. Some people have a tattoo with a meaningful phrase that helped them through difficult times.

- Especially over the last decades, tattoos have become an expression of individuality and an extension of personal style. Images to confirm originality are often bold to make a strong statement.

- Many rebellious teenagers and young adults express their independence from their parents through daring tattoos.

- Also, people with scars or birthmarks have a tattoo to hide the scar. A young mother might prefer to have her baby's name tattooed on a stretch mark, or an accident victim might choose to hide a burn wound in this way.

Public perceptions about tattoos have changed drastically during the past two decades. Previously, people with tattoos were often judged. Today, tattoos are much more acceptable, and many young people have tattoos. However, bold and big tattoos, especially on the face and neck, evoke negative comments.

How Is a Tattoo Done?

The information in this section is not meant to prevent you from getting a tattoo, although the process and possible side effects may sound scary. Knowledge about the tattoo process explains why it is so difficult to remove, expensive, and often requires several sessions over a long period.

Having a tattoo can be painful because it is a seriously invasive procedure. There are different types of tattoo machines: a machine with electromagnetic coils and magnets, a rotary machine with a spinning action, or a pneumatic or pressurised machine.

They all lift an armature bar and bring it forcefully down to penetrate the skin between 50 and 3,000 times per minute (MeDermis Laser Clinic, 2022). A group of needles attached to the bar repeatedly punch the skin. The needles, made of steel, nickel, or chrome, vary in thickness from 0.25 to 0.40 mm, but the standard needle is 0.35 mm (Barber DST, 2022). However, modern magnum needles are thinner and can punch the skin up to 6,000 times a minute (Saved Tattoo, 2022).

The tattoo artist controls the machine by a handheld stainless steel tube, which is easily sterilised. When the needles are lifted, it draws the ink in.

The tattoo artist does your image pretty much as you drew a picture as a toddler, except that they use needles, not crayons. First, the outlines are punched with 'liners', grouped in a tight bundle. Secondly, the artist does the shading with 'shaders', which are also grouped in a circle or a fan form.

When the needles are tapped into the skin, the skin surface is broken and the needles penetrate right through the epidermis into the dermis. The needle points form a hole and release the ink into the hole. However, this hole is not empty but filled with macrophages and fibroblasts, skin cells previously mentioned. To recap, macrophages are white blood or immune cells responsible for killing microorganisms and helping the cyclic removal of dead cells. Fibroblasts form the skin's connective tissue, produce collagen, and help give structure to the face.

Furthermore, to emphasise how difficult it is to remove a tattoo, the needles penetrate the skin about 3 cm deep. As said earlier, it is a painful process, and especially areas with many nerve endings experience severe pain. Luckily, the forearms, stomach, and outer thighs have fewer nerve endings and are slightly less sensitive.

Tattoo Ink

The ink stays in this little hole permanently, colouring your skin to form your unique image. Tattoos fade slightly over the years because the body recognises the ink as foreign matter and tries to get rid of it. Unfortunately, ink is quite obstinate and does not go willingly or fast.

The ink contains a carrier such as glycerin, water, isopropyl alcohol, or witch hazel. These are safe, but unscrupulous manufacturers may use dangerous liquids such as antifreeze, formaldehyde, or methanol.

Tattoo ink needs a colourant, and there are more than 200 types to choose from. Many tattoo inks contain heavy metals such as antimony, beryllium, lead, cobalt-nickel, chromium, or arsenic. Manufacturers also add adhesives, binding agents, and preservatives.

Some colours are more prone to cause allergies: red, then blue, green, and black. Modern tattoo artists use animal and vegan inks, which are not necessarily safe. They may be contaminated or cause allergies; therefore, regulation is necessary to make tattoo ink and permanent make-up safe for consumers.

Regulation

In the U.K., tattoo ink producers are not yet under a legal obligation to reveal their ingredients, but authorities are looking into regulation procedures. Authorities warn that some ingredients might have hazardous substances (UK REACH, 2021).

The European Union has restricted the use of certain chemicals in tattoo ink since January 2022 (UK Reach, 2021).

The Food and Drug Administration (FDA) of the United States issued a safety advisory in May 2015 about contaminated tattoo products (FDA, 2022). However, the United States tattoo industry is still largely unregulated in 2022. In the United States, tattoo ink is classified as a cosmetic product, and ingredients must be listed on the labels (Chung, 2022).

What Can Go Wrong?

Unfortunately, several things can go wrong:

- The wound can become infected.

- The skin might have an immediate allergic reaction.

- A delayed allergic reaction, even years afterward, is possible.

- In rare cases, a tattoo blowout develops, a condition where the ink spreads into the fat layer underneath the skin, and the design is distorted.

- The needle can puncture a blood vein, and the ink will enter your bloodstream. Usually, the body breaks it down.

Why Do People Have Tattoo Regret?

A Texas Tech University study found that more people approach dermatologists to have their tattoos removed. Most are white, unmarried young women with a college degree (Colihan, 2008).

The reasons given are a strange mix of 'just decided to do it', embarrassment, negative impact on body image, not suitable for a new profession, does not suit clothes, and to a lesser extent, stigmatisation (Colihan, 2oo8). The first reason, 'just decided to do it', tells a somewhat complicated backstory. What prompted these young women to get the unwelcome tattoo in the first palace? Was it a rash decision? And under what circumstances was it done? Why is it now haunting them?

If you consider having a tattoo, it might be a good idea not to rush into a tattoo parlour. Consider the following situations for why women like you will want a tattoo removed in a few years:

- An ex's name is the most common reason to remove a tattoo. Back to Johnny Depp: He had 'Wynona Forever' tattooed on his right shoulder and, after their breakup, changed it to 'Wino Forever': 'actually a bit more accurate', Depp told *Playboy* (Jones, 2014).

- Tattoos done during a night of drinking often are an acute embarrassment. Dermatologists report frequent calls from distressed young women after a rash decision to have a funny or downright stupid tattoo done while not thinking straight.

- Trends come and go, and women tire of trendy tattoos quickly. For example, during the 1980s, barbed wire and tribal tattoos were immensely popular, and now people find them meaningless. Dermatologists also notice that young women regret trendy tattoos featured on Pinterest and Instagram that are no longer fashionable. They recommend that women overthink an idea for a tattoo for at least a few months before having it done.

- Flowers, butterflies, and bird tattoos done during youth often become an embarrassment later in life, and dermatologists frequently have to remove these images at a great cost a few years later.

- If you are considering a professional career, think twice before you have a tattoo done on the fingers, hands, or ankles. In some set-ups, visible tattoos are not tolerated, and they might become an embarrassment to you.

- People mostly regret tattoos on the face, upper arms, upper back, hips, and butt.

How Are Tattoos Removed?

The body's immune system cannot destroy tattoo ink pigments in the dermis, as they are too large. Laser removal helps the body to naturally remove the pigment, as it breaks up the pigments into minute particles.

The shallow ink deposits are removed more quickly than those trapped in the dermis. The laser heats the skin, and the pigment absorbs the heat, which breaks down the pigment. Some ink types only disintegrate at very high temperatures, which will cause burn wounds and scar the skin. Modern lasers use intense heat waves in very short bursts, long enough to heat the pigment but not scar the skin.

Black is the easiest colour to remove, as black pigment reacts to all laser wavelengths, thus breaking up rapidly. The more colours and the darker the tattoo, the longer it will take to remove it. A bold and dark image might need regular treatments over a period, and even then, it might not be completely erased.

Your skin has to recover after each session for a few weeks. It could thus take months to remove a tattoo. Laser treatment is not relaxing, and you might find it highly uncomfortable or even painful. The dermatologist will apply a numbing cream and instructions on aftercare. Some doctors recommend breathing techniques during the treatment. Others will hold a lively conversation while the patient plays with a squeezy ball, which confirms: Laser treatment to remove tattoo ink is not an easy process.

Unfortunately, up to date, it is the only method to remove tattoos.

Quick Reminder

The skin is a powerful storyteller; tattoos tell the world what or who is important to you.

The tattoo machine uses needles to puncture the skin right into the dermis, about 3 mm deep.

It can punch the skin thousands of times per minute, an invasive and painful process.

The ink is released in the dermis between cells vital to skin health: fibroblasts and macrophages.

Infection, skin allergies, and several other risks are possible; some people develop an allergic reaction years afterward.

Dermatologists report increasing requests for tattoo removal; the most common is getting rid of an ex's name.

Only repeated laser treatments can eliminate or fade the tattoo by releasing high-energy waves.

It can take months to remove a tattoo as the heat breaks down the ink into small particles for the body to remove.

Chapter 12:
Stubborn Cellulite

Merriam-Webster defines cellulite as deposits of subcutaneous fat within fibrous connective tissue (as in the thighs, hips, and buttocks) that give a puckered and dimpled appearance to the skin surface.

The dictionary's compilers wisely did not mention that mostly women have cellulite, but unfortunately it is true. More women than men have cellulite: Some sources estimate that 80 to 90% of women have cellulite compared to 10% of men (Cleveland, 2021).

Cellulite does not discriminate between over- or underweight women. Even the skinniest of women can have cellulite. Still, cellulite is often more visible in overweight or obese people. Some women are lucky, and their cellulite is only visible if they pinch the skin between their fingers. Others show cellulite even when sitting down, while others show cellulite only when standing.

However, most women agree that cellulite is stubborn: unwilling to go, unattractive, and unwelcome.

Why Do Women Have More Cellulite?

Research on the causes of cellulite is inconclusive, but experts agree cellulite has to do with the fibrous band that connects the skin to the underlying muscle. They believe this fibrous band tightens, pulls the skin down, and the underlying fat is pushed upward between the bands, causing small pockets of fat that look like orange skin.

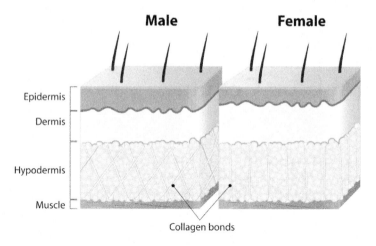

Male **Female**

Epidermis

Dermis

Hypodermis

Muscle

Collagen bonds

One theory is that women are more prone to cellulite as the skin structure differs in men and women. In men, the bands connecting the hypodermis or subcutaneous fat layer run crisscross, while these bands run parallel in women.

Another theory is that oestrogen causes cellulite. This theory is supported by the fact that cellulite usually appears during puberty and pregnancy.

People with darker skin are less likely to show cellulite, another benefit of having darker skin.

Can Cellulite Be Removed?

Unfortunately, cellulite cannot be removed entirely. However, it can be improved by healthy living – a combination of diet, exercise, salon, and medical treatments. Most treatments are only temporary and must be repeated regularly to keep cellulite under control.

A holistic approach to combat cellulite is the only real solution. You must live healthily – cutting out processed foods and sugars and exercising regularly for the rest of your life. Also, choose an affordable treatment from the list below to complement your healthy lifestyle, and you will see results within months.

Your cellulite will not magically disappear, though. Over time, you will be healthier, your body more toned, and your general appearance and cellulite will improve.

Lifestyle Choices to Combat Cellulite

As a first step in combatting cellulite, you have to live healthily. You can get the most expensive treatment available, but it will be in vain if you treat your body with disregard. Eating correctly and exercising regularly will enhance the treatments below. A healthy lifestyle is discussed in the previous chapter and is the point of departure for any woman struggling with cellulite.

Diet

The following are especially good for the skin and, therefore, also for cellulite:

- Fruits: Grapefruit has high amounts of vitamin C, which burns fats, stimulates the metabolism, and thus causes weight loss. Furthermore, it helps with hydration. Fruit and vegetables have antioxidants, phytonutrients, and bioflavonoids, which are vital for healthy skin. Consider supplements with coffee, Biloba, and grape-seed extract. Add a slice of lemon to your water for a generally healthier body: improved hydration, removing toxins and vitamin C.

- Vegetables: Asparagus is rich in folic acid, which reduces stress. Stress is a recognised factor in fat storage. Folic acid also helps with blood circulation, which removes toxins. Beetroot is high in polyphenols, while avocados and dark green, leafy vegetables provide antioxidants. Try to eat vegetables raw or baked to prevent nutrient loss through boiling.

- Herbs: Coriander contains vitamins and boosts the immune system. Furthermore, coriander removes toxic heavy metals from the system and improves the appearance of cellulite. Parsley also contains vitamins to improve general skin quality and helps to flush toxins from the body. Many people use parsley only as a garnish to finish off a dish. In the Middle East, parsley is chopped, and large quantities are added to salads, smoothies, and sandwiches. Whether ginger is a herb or a spice does not matter: Ginger improves blood flow, bringing fresh oxygen to the skin and at the same time removing toxins quicker. Ginger has medical properties, but if you wish to flush the toxins from your body, have ginger in your tea or add it to your dishes.

- Nuts and seeds are high in Omega-3 fatty acids, invaluable in keeping the skin cell membrane healthy and slowing ageing. It also fights inflammation. Flaxseeds are a rich source of Omega-3 fatty acids, but they are so small that they cannot be chewed properly. Use flaxseed oil, eat them grounded in cereals, or add them to a smoothie. Another option is to soak flaxseeds before adding them to dishes, as they will digest better.

- Grains provide fibre and are vital for a healthy gut. A well-functioning digestive system gets rid of toxins quicker and will improve your skin and cellulite appearance. Furthermore, grains promote cardiac health and blood circulation. Buckwheat is pseudo-grain, not a proper grain, but its seeds function like grain. It contains fibre, has proteins, and is rich in vitamin B. It also contains lysine, an amino acid important in collagen production. Buckwheat is excellent for fighting cellulite, as it helps in many ways to build the skin and remove toxins to improve cellulite.

Foods to avoid

Avoid sugar, processed foods, sauces, white bread, and pastries if you want to keep your skin healthy. Sugar comes from highly refined grains, and sugars and processed foods are packed with sugar. Sugar breaks down elastin and collagen, the main proteins in your skin. As collagen and elastin are destroyed, the skin sags, wrinkles, and dries. Your skin ages while the fat builds up underneath and cellulite becomes more prominent.

Sugar also causes uncontrolled inflammation, contributing to acne and other skin conditions.

Exercise

Exercise alone will not remove cellulite, but it is essential to your holistic approach to keeping it under control. Exercise in combination with an improved diet usually contributes to weight loss, resulting in toned muscles and a leaner body that will improve the appearance of dimpled pockets of fat.

Exercise strengthens and tightens muscles under the skin and thus also under the cellulite areas. A combination of strength training and cardio gives the best results. Cardio exercises strengthen the heart and lung function, which increases blood flow and oxygen supply to the areas affected by cellulite. Running, cycling, walking, and swimming are excellent cardio exercises.

Strength exercises such as resistance bands and Pilates build muscles and even help burn calories when you rest. You can do targeted strength training to strengthen the muscles in your thighs or upper arms and do cardio exercises for general fitness.

Don't expect overnight improvement, but in two to three months of exercise and healthy living, you will look better, and cellulite will be less visible.

Medical and Salon Treatments

Topical Retinol and Other Applications

Many topical creams and lotions claim to break down fat. Others contain vitamins, minerals, and herbal extracts, and regular massage could reduce cellulite visibility. Retinol creams might work, but not enough scientific evidence is available yet.

Acoustic Wave Therapy

This treatment for kidney stones is now also used for cellulite. High-energy waves break kidney stones into minute bits that can be passed with urine. It is a non-invasive treatment, and you can have it twice a week. Some sources say cellulite visibility will improve within two to six months; others are still unconvinced that it helps.

Cryolipolysis

Freezing is a non-invasive procedure that freezes and kills the fat cells. The body naturally gets rid of the dead cells. It is usually done for body contouring but is also used to get rid of cellulite, as the body has to remove the dead cells. Results are only visible after three to four months.

Deep Massage

Massage is the stalwart treatment for cellulite, as it increases blood flow and reduces fluid build-up. Mechanical devices using low-pressure rollers knead the skin between two spinning rollers. According to the manufacturers, it breaks up the connective tissue. However, the effect is only short-lived, and some experts believe the skin can become stretched and slack.

Laser Treatment

A laser beam releases heat in three directions to improve cellulite. Laser treatment often includes other treatment options such as massage, liposuction, and light therapy. It is a comprehensive treatment to liquefy fat, reduce fluid retention, cut connective tissue to loosen the puckering, boost collagen production, and increase blood flow.

Treatments should be repeated annually for maintenance.

Radiofrequency-Assisted Lipolysis

It is a minimally invasive treatment done with a handheld device. Radiofrequency energy and suction are combined to melt and remove fat. It is further combined with laser and massage. It causes bruising but shows promising results.

Mesotherapy

Chemicals injected into the fat layer below the skin are supposed to break down the fat, but the risk of allergies and infection is relatively high. Most doctors do not recommend it, as patients report several side effects such as redness, swelling, tenderness, and changes to the skin.

Liposuction

Some dermatologists suggest liposuction for removing excess fat, but the treatment is not always successful. Some doctors combine liposuction with laser treatment. It is important to know that liposuction is invasive, and you will need some downtime to recover.

Ultrasound liposculpting is relatively new, but unfortunately, not enough scientific evidence is available yet.

Subcision

It is a minimally invasive needle treatment, during which the doctor breaks the connective tissue with a needle and the fat smooths out.

In a more advanced technique, the doctor uses a handheld device. A tiny blade cuts the connective tissue to release the fat bundles. The device is vacuum-controlled to ensure the precise depth of the cutting.

The dermatologist can treat about 2o to 30 fat dimples during a session of about one hour (Axell, 2020). Results are visible after about one month and can last for two to three years.

Spa Treatments

Spa technicians use a combination of different treatments.

Ionithermie Treatment

The area is covered by a mixture of clay and algae. Electrodes are attached and then wrapped in plastics. A mild current is applied to reduce cellulite. Unfortunately, there is no scientific evidence to support the success of this treatment. The treatment causes discomfort but is not painful.

Vacuum-Assisted Tissue Release

The treatment is based on traditional cupping treatment and is called endermology. A vacuum device lifts the skin and massages it. However, there is no evidence that the treatment works.

Traditional Treatments

Ginkgo Biloba

Ginkgo biloba leaves are traditionally used in Chinese medicine to increase blood flow. It opens the micro-capillaries and strengthens the vessel walls. It helps to bring fresh blood with oxygen, which accelerates the breakdown of fat and releases fatty acids.

Grape-Seed Extract

Grape-seed oil also promotes blood flow and strengthens the artery walls. They contain polyphenols and antioxidants and improve skin health.

Cupping

Cupping is an ancient method from China and the Middle East. Traditionally, ceramic cups were heated and placed on the area. When it is pulled off, it pulls the blood and lymph capillaries to the surface, smoothing the skin. The healer also massaged the area with oils to improve blood circulation.

Unfortunately, research has not confirmed this theory. Modern salons use a vacuum-assisted method based on ancient cupping practices. See above.

Dry Brushing

Dry brushing is a traditional method of massaging the skin with a dry brush. The bristles help remove dead skin cells and leave the skin looking fresh. It has several benefits. It unclogs pores and improves blood and lymph circulation, leaving the skin glowing. It stimulates the nervous system and energises. Unfortunately, dry brushing does not help to diminish cellulite.

However, it can help the skin look better, which does improve the general appearance.

Cellulite and Cellulitis

Cellulite and cellulitis might sound similar, but they are not related. Cellulitis is a bacterial infection that occurs most often on infected skin. People get it mostly on their feet and legs.

Initially, it causes redness, swelling, and pain. The skin appears pitted with blisters. If untreated, it can become serious. Infection might spread to the blood, joints, bones, and even heart valves' lining. The patient should take antibiotics as soon as possible.

Quick Reminder

Women are more prone to cellulite; few men have cellulite.

The cause is uncertain, but presumably, the fibrous band connecting the skin to the fat layer underneath plays a role in pressing down and forcing the fat upward between the bands to give the puckered effect.

There is no permanent cure for cellulite but a holistic approach.

A healthy diet, regular cardio, and strength exercises help tone the body and help with weight loss, improving cellulite's appearance.

Several medical practices can temporarily improve cellulite but have to be repeated for maintenance.

Despite similarly sounding names, cellulitis is not related to cellulite.

Cellulitis is serious, and medical care is necessary.

Part 3: Beauty: Past, Present, and Future

Chapter 13:
Skincare Myths

To love beauty is to see light.

Victor Hugo, the author of *Les Misérables,* wished for the miserables of the world to see the light. On a somewhat different level, women should see the light and look past the beauty trade's 101 myths.

The question is: How far can one believe the labels, the media, and the urban legends about skincare? Women often consult Dr. Google, but unfortunately, Dr. Google does not have all the answers. One writer swears that eye cream is an absolute must; the other says the skin around the eye does not differ from the skin on the rest of the face, thus no special cream is necessary. It's chaos for the average consumer who does not know whom to believe.

A reliable trick to get the truth is to check who the expert is. Who is swearing by an eye cream? Is it a dermatologist who sells skincare products? Or a dermatologist who is not involved in retail?

Beware of meaningless marketing terms that might manipulate you into believing a product has exceptional qualities. You will find a list of beauty buzzwords later in this chapter.

Media Myths

Misleading Marketing and Advertising

Marketing is a broad term and includes the product name, labelling, packaging, and, last but not least, advertising material about the product.

Cosmetic advertisers promote products cleverly. They target emotions; a woman might not even have thought of buying a moisturiser but seeing the ad creates a need to look and feel better about herself. Most women know advertising can be calculated and misleading but often are emotional, not objective, about personal issues and want to look as good as the woman on the billboard.

Unethical advertisers play on consumer emotions. They often make unsubstantiated promises about their products to boost sales. Marketers are aware of the human need to look better, feel better, and be accepted by others. They sometimes exploit these emotions and give false hope to people with skin problems. Beware of half-truths, false claims, and vague information.

To make matters worse, there is no escaping from advertisements: One hears the ad on TV and sees it on the billboards. It promises to relieve those worrying issues: dryness, fine lines, acne, etc. It's only human to want to improve your looks.

Keep an eye open for specific patterns and buzzwords, and you will soon learn to distinguish between empty marketing promises and creams that indeed can help retain the moisture in your skin.

Social Media

Traditionally, advertisers used the media – billboards, printed media, and TV – to reach the consumer. However, during the past few years, they started using social media to track consumers' interests to promote their products. Their promotional messages are often personalised to address the individual's perceived needs.

More Marketing Tricks

Misleading marketing does not stop at advertising.

Unscrupulous companies have many tricks to fool consumers. One such scheme is to repack cheap products in fancy small tubes to fit your bag. The content might be the same as the pot in the local supermarket, but their presentation suggests they are exclusively produced from high-end ingredients.

Another trick is using before and after photos. At first glance, the improvement is impressive. However, chances are good that the images are carefully staged. Usually, the model wears no make-up in the first photo but is professionally groomed for the after-image. For all we know, the model might have had several other treatments contributing to the different striking look. Furthermore, pictures are very easily photoshopped to enhance their appearance.

Decypher the Labels

The product's price is often the deciding factor in buying a specific product. Checking the label can help you decide between an affordable and expensive cream. The more expensive product might be better because it contains a particular ingredient. The opposite can also be true: A cheaper product might have the same ingredients.

The label is often an obvious giveaway of counterfeit and inferior products: Spelling mistakes, typos, and poor printing are red flags. If the presentation is unprofessional, the product might also be suspect.

Look at the label very carefully. There are several sections of information besides the product's name: product purpose, manufacturer, retailer, brand name and address, expiry date, and then, in much finer print, the ingredients. If in doubt, go to the brand's official website and ensure the label information is authentic. Unscrupulous marketers often use names similar-sounding to well-established and trusted brands to mislead consumers.

Firstly, the product's purpose is a good starting point. Night cream, eye cream, sunscreen? If the information sounds too good to be true, it probably is not true. (Below are some examples of misleading marketing terms.)

Secondly, where was it manufactured and by whom? A product from a reputable company must adhere to the country of origin's high standards. Can you trust a product from an undeclared place of origin?

Thirdly, go to the ingredient list. Look for the ingredients discussed in this book. Look for the ingredient that can target your skin's needs. You will often find that the more affordable product contains many of the same ingredients as the expensive one.

Empty Buzzwords and Wild Promises

Absorbed and active deep in the skin

Claims about a product's ability to penetrate and work deep in the skin to heal or stimulate regeneration must be taken with a pinch of salt. Another urban myth is that the skin absorbs 60% of topical creams. The stratum corneum forms an impenetrable barrier, and cosmetic products cannot penetrate the skin to be absorbed. If creams cannot penetrate the skin, they cannot reach the deeper layers. However, this does not imply that skin products are useless: They work in many other ways.

Active ingredients

Active ingredients are discussed in Chapter 3. To recap, they are not substances but biologically active ingredients such as glycolic acid, alpha-hydroxy acid (AHAs), retinol and vitamin C. They biologically change some aspects of the skin cells. Although highly rated in skincare, it is not always better to buy a product with a high percentage of an active ingredient. The active ingredient's activity in the skin is not necessarily better when highly concentrated: It depends on the pH level and might be more effective at a low pH level.

Age-defying and anti-ageing

These are two overused marketing claims, usually with little scientific backing. At most, the product can protect the skin barrier and prevent moisture loss. A cream alone can hardly stop ageing: Several other factors play a role in preventing premature ageing.

Alcohol and alcohol-free

Many skincare products contain alcohol, and alcohol is not necessarily bad. Fatty and aromatic alcohols have positive roles in skincare. Fatty alcohol is a thickening agent that combines with the moisture in the stratum corneum to prevent moisture loss. Also, minute quantities of aromatic alcohol give a pleasant flavour and usually do not affect the skin. However, women with highly sensitive skin should avoid aromatic alcohol in their products.

Also, simple alcohol can be problematic in high concentrations. It weakens the skin barrier and contributes to dryness. If you suspect a product dries your skin, check the label for simple alcohol under the names isopropyl and denatured alcohol.

Animal testing

For a very long time, it was standard procedure to test products on animals before testing them on humans. Animals suffered incredible pain. Rabbits, guinea pigs, hamsters, mice, and rats were exposed to torturous laboratory practices to produce lipsticks and luxurious creams.

Fortunately, global resistance exposed animal testing. Many countries have since banned animal testing. Check for the leaping bunny logo if you don't want to support the movement. More than 700 companies across the globe have the leaping bunny certification, indicating that they do not test their products on animals (One Planet, 2018).

Chemical-free

Chemical-free is another misused term that influences the consumer's natural adversity to any chemical substances. It is a misplaced perception that chemicals are bad. The human body is made up of water, and water is a chemical. The body's main other building blocks are also chemical elements. The same goes for skincare products: They all contain chemicals, and a general term such as 'chemical-free' means little.

Of course, there are many toxic chemicals, and one such chemical is formaldehyde, often used in hair products. Avoid it at all costs, as it can cause severe diseases such as cancer.

Clinical trials/clinically proven

The term 'clinical trial' is often misused to imply that the product is based on medical research. A clinical trial is a scientific study under strict control and according to a specific scientific design and method. A clinical trial is monitored, audited, and the analyses must be published in a report or academic article.

Cosmetic houses often do a consumer trial during which a selected group of women use the product for a specific period. The women then complete a questionnaire to report their observations and personal assessments. It is not a controlled medical study based on scientific findings. Brands often use these consumer trials not so much to get feedback on the product but as a promotion gimmick. Remember, the product has already been developed and is ready for the market when the consumer trial is run.

Dermatologist recommended/dermatologist tested

When dermatologists test products, they do several repeat insult patch tests (RIPT) to check for possible allergic reactions. The repeat insult patch test is a well-respected method recognised by experts and the global cosmetic industry.

However, dermatologist-recommended means that a dermatologist has been paid to approve the product. To add insult to injury, the term is often used very loosely without even the name of a dermatologist. Check the brand's website if you are uncertain about the credentials of any claim.

Green and sustainable products

Most consumers believe green products are good for the planet. Green is often used interchangeably with organic or natural products; therefore, eco-friendly. They are manufactured from sustainable sources and without any pollution during the manufacturing.

Are the specific products indeed green? But what does it mean? Is there any evidence of organic registration? Does it have legal certification?

Unfortunately, many so-called green skincare products contain one or another form of petroleum generated by the petrochemical industry – notorious for pollution.

If you suspect the term green is just a marketing gimmick, check for the following unhealthy ingredients:

- *Formaldehyde,* as discussed above, can harm the environment.

- *BHA and BHT* are synthetic antioxidants and are often used as preservatives in lipsticks.

- *Coal tar dyes or p-phenylenediamine* are colourants and pose a risk of cancer.

- Deodorants may contain *aluminium* linked to a risk for breast cancer.

- Nail products often use the solvent *dibutyl phthalate (DBP),* which is toxic for pregnant women (Acme-Hardesty, n.d.).

Also, check whether the wrappings and containers are recyclable, often a sign of a retailer that cares about the environment.

Hypoallergenic

Hypoallergenic implies the product is free of substances that might cause allergies. A respectable company will be hesitant to make this claim, as irritations and allergies can be caused by numerous synthetic and natural ingredients such as perfumes, preservatives, or other substances. Furthermore, health authorities have not defined the term 'hypoallergenic'; thus, the meaning is unclear. It is a marketing slogan when not backed by reliable scientific proof.

Non-comedogenic

Non-comedogenic implies that the product won't clog the pores. As with 'hypoallergenic', there is not an official definition of the properties of a non-comedogenic product. Again, it is a vague claim that might or might not work for an individual. It would be unwise to buy a specific product based on a claim that it is non-comedogenic. Read the chapter on acne, identify your problem, and consult a dermatologist if you can't find an effective over-the-counter product.

Preservative-free

Skincare ingredients need preservatives to prevent bacteria and mould growth. They would go off in about three weeks if they didn't contain preservatives.

The European Union has banned the terms 'chemical-free', 'toxin-free', and 'chemical-free' from advertisements and labels as they can mislead customers.

Parabens are the most commonly used, and at least one expert says they are not harmful in small doses of less than 1% (Frey, 2021). Other scientific studies found that parabens have dangerous health risks and are bad for the environment. Look out for parabens with the following names: butylparaben, methylparaben, and propylparaben. Chapter 3 discusses parabens in more detail.

Fortunately, there are healthier alternatives for parabens: phenoxyethanol, benzyl alcohol, sodium benzoate, potassium sorbate, ethylhexyl, glycerin, and others. Don't be scared of these weird chemical terms, or even try to remember them, but check before buying a new product.

'60% fewer wrinkles in x weeks'

A precise percentage or number in any ad is usually misleading. What is the marketer's definition of a wrinkle? A fine line, a deep groove? How were those wrinkles measured at the beginning and end of the trial?

'Youthful skin within x weeks'

Ask yourself: Can any cream give you back your youthful skin? Why are millions of women still struggling with dry skin and wrinkles despite using these creams?

Myths About Ingredients and Products

Consumers insist on environmentally friendly products more than ever, but misleading advertising and misconceptions are still rife. Look at products and their ingredients critically to ensure that advertising does not take you for a ride.

Natural and Organic Products

Natural Products

Natural is not always better, and all-natural products are not necessarily good. Many natural products are not regulated, and you have no guarantee that all the ingredients are natural.

There are numerous misconceptions about what natural products are, their benefit in skincare, and their sustainability.

Essential oils are examples of natural products. Essential oils are distilled from plants' flowers, leaves, roots, or fruit. It is the essence of the plant in an undiluted form. Essential oils are regularly used in most skincare products and are known for their healing properties. The mere name evokes images of lavender fields or sweet-smelling roses.

But essential oils directly applied to the skin can irritate and burn. They need a base or carrier oil before applying it to the skin. The carrier oil plays a vital role in absorbing the essential oil. A too heavy carrier oil might neutralise the effectiveness of the essential oil.

Not all products advertised as natural are entirely natural. Some ingredients may be plant-derived but are processed and chemically modified in a laboratory. The process does not necessarily make them less effective, but the information is incorrect. Why use incorrect information if the product is good?

Beware of the claim that a natural product is gentle. Just because it comes from nature does not mean it is gentle and good for the skin. Some natural products can be harsh and burn the skin.

Organic Products

Natural ingredients are not necessarily organic. Not even so-called organic products are always organic.

Organic products are natural ingredients without chemicals, fertilisers, pesticides, antibiotics, parabens, or genetically modified organisms (GMOs). Organic skincare products may not contain any synthetic ingredients.

How is this monitored? Farm markets with organic vegetables, eggs, and meat have become very popular worldwide. But are these products genuinely organic? Or has organic become a marketing term that implies the consumer can buy directly from the farmer and skip the retailer?

Most countries regulate organic products. In the U.S.A., the Department of Agriculture gives a seal of approval if at least 95% of a product contains organic ingredients (USDA Organic, 2022). In the U.K., organic farmers must register with an organic control body. Certification depends on regular inspections and close adherence to regulations. It provides peace of mind and protects the consumer (Gov.UK, 2020).

Sustainability and Packaging

The beauty industry is vast, and its impact on the environment is disturbing. The industry is notorious for its negative footprint on nature. Apart from testing on animals, production waste, and energy consumption, packaging is a significant concern.

According to reports from Zero Waste Week, 120 billion packaging pieces are used in the beauty industry every year (Okafor, 2022). Assuming those pretty boxes and containers land in the refuse bin, it amounts to unacceptable levels.

The most disturbing aspect is that the pretty boxes and wrappings are purely decorative, skilful marketing to manipulate the consumer to buy into 'luxury'. Unfortunately, consumers are as guilty as the manufacturers. We love the beautiful packaging but often throw it in the bin without a second thought.

That brings another dilemma to the fore. Recycling has become trendy over the last decade. Many of us sort our refuse into different containers, proud that we can contribute to a greener society. Unfortunately, beauty packaging is not easy to recycle. Manufacturers combine paper, glass, and plastic, making it impractical to sort and only suitable for the landfill site.

Toxins and plastics end up in the ocean, devastatingly affecting marine life and water resources.

Sustainability and Natural Biospheres

You might think it is better to use a product containing natural products. Quite the opposite is true, though. Often, natural resources are not sustainable, and natural biospheres are destroyed in the harvesting of products. Unethical companies use the term 'natural' to lure you into thinking that natural is sustainable.

Palm oil is such an example. You might be surprised at how many products contain palm oil. Harvesting the oil destroys palm forests at an alarming rate, and animals living in these forests die with the trees.

It is time that we start caring about the environmental impact of the products. Let the company know if you like a product but object to taking off three or four layers of packaging. One voice will not make much difference, but 20 or 100 women airing their concerns might radically change the industry.

Synthetic Products

What are synthetic ingredients, and why do they have such a bad name? Synthetic ingredients are made in a laboratory and are thus manmade versions of natural ingredients.

One such example is hyaluronic acid: This key ingredient was initially harvested from fermented bacteria of – wait for it – rooster combs. Scientists then replicated the exact composition in the laboratory. Other examples include synthetic vitamin C.

Synthetic ingredients usually have a longer shelf life than natural ones, making them more profitable and sustainable. Natural ingredients are harvested at a considerable cost, and farming equipment like tractors and harvesting machines are anything but eco-friendly. Remember that only a small percentage of natural products are farmed organically. Most farmers still use fertilisers, pesticides, and growth hormones of some kind.

In short, many synthetic ingredients are produced cheaper and have a smaller environmental footprint. Health authorities regulate their production, and they are safe to use. Sometimes the answer to saving the planet does not lie in going entirely green but in making informed decisions.

Urban Myths About Daily Skincare

Necessary or Not?

Eye Creams

The eye cream debate is ongoing. According to Dr Fayne Frey, New York board-certified clinical and surgical dermatologist, the skin around the eye and on the cheekbones is the same (Frey, 2021).

Other experts say an eye cream suitable for your skin may help with dark circles and puffiness. Still others say eye creams containing caffeine can reduce inflammation in the area. They say the ideal combination for an eye cream is caffeine, hyaluronic acid, and retinol (Forbes, 2021).

Toners

Toners dry the skin because they are loaded with alcohol. It might have been true of old-fashioned toners, but modern toners contain much-needed acids, glycerin, antioxidants, and even anti-inflammatories. They remove the last bits of cleanser and leave the skin moist; the ideal condition for the moisturiser to hydrate the top layer of keratinocytes and the minute spaces between them. Apply your moisturiser immediately after the toner to benefit most.

These Myths Can Be Dangerous

Sunscreen

Nearly every chapter in this book mentions sunscreen. It is no wonder that many dermatologists view sunscreen as vital and even the most critical product in skincare. Despite all the information on skin cancer and photoaging, there are still numerous misconceptions about sunscreen. Read Chapter 5 on hyperpigmentation for more detail on UV radiation and sunscreen SPF.

Please take note:

- Spray tanning does not protect the skin against sunburn.

- A spray tan is a colourant and nothing more.

- A base tan does not protect against UV radiation. It is a misconception that can do serious harm.

- Sunbeds are not safe; they are as dangerous as the sun itself.

- Always wear sunscreen: whether summer, winter, or cloudy.

- Wear sunscreen even if you wear other products containing SPF.

Water

Drinking water is necessary to keep the body hydrated, but the skin does not absorb water. Neither is it true that water can remove wrinkles. However, dehydration is dangerous, and the body, and eventually the skin, will suffer.

You cannot cure dry skin by drinking water. A moisturiser that seals the skin barrier and prevents further moisture loss is the solution for dry skin. Chapter 8 on ageing discusses the difference between dry and dehydrated skin. You will also find a simple finger test to determine whether your skin is dehydrated.

Skincare Myths

Expensive equals better

Expensive does not always equal better. The expense part often lies in packaging and marketing costs. Compare the packaging of an expensive cream to that of regular cream. The costly one probably comes in an uncommonly shaped jar, which is expensive to produce. Furthermore, the pot is wrapped in several different wrappings. Also, the box is often textured, either velvety or super smooth, sometimes even with gold lettering. The expense is in the packaging, not necessarily in the content of the product.

Exfoliate every day

You must exfoliate the skin regularly is another myth that can be harmful. The skin renews itself about once a month. Over-exfoliating the skin can harm the barrier and expose the skin to sunburn, pollution, and infections.

Retinoids are only necessary after 50

Retinoid is a vitamin A derivative, vital in stimulating cell turnover in the skin. In the 20s, the production of collagen and elastin starts slowing down, and retinoids stimulate the rejuvenation of skin cells. Retinoids boost collagen production and unclog pores. The earlier you begin, the better.

Don't moisturise oily skin

Oily skin needs moisturising as much as dry skin. Sebum, which makes the skin oily, is waxy but ineffective in retaining hydration. Moisturisers on the stratum corneum seal the surface to keep the skin hydrated. Dry and dehydrated skin looks old and is more prone to infections and inflammation.

Don't wash your skin in the morning

You have to clean your face in the morning. You might think your face is clean because you have not been outside and exposed to dirt or sweat. Nonetheless, your linen might not be squeaky clean, and pollution particles are everywhere in the air. Clean your face gently morning and night without robbing it of its natural moisturisers.

Cleaning the skin with make-up wipes is enough

Make-up wipes are not suitable for cleaning the face. They are designed to break down make-up particles. You must clean your face to remove the dirt and bacteria from your skin.

Bad hygiene causes acne

Bad hygiene does not cause acne. Washing your face more often will not heal acne. An overproduction of sebum causes acne. It is essential to determine why the sebaceous glands are producing too much sebum and address the real cause of acne. Hygiene is obviously vital, but bad hygiene is not the reason for acne.

Quick Reminder

Unfortunately, unscrupulous marketers and advertisements purposely mislead consumers. But labels on products from reliable brands help consumers choose the right ingredients.

Read and understand the labels before buying a product.

Make sure you recognise meaningless terminology some marketers use to influence the buyer.

Natural products are not always entirely natural. They often contain synthetic ingredients.

Natural products are not always kinder to the environment; their cultivation can have a significant carbon footprint.

Natural does not necessarily equal organic.

Organic farmers must be registered and adhere to strict regulations. They are not allowed to use chemicals in crop production.

Synthetic products are not necessarily harmful to the consumer or the environment. Their production is often cheaper and more sustainable than natural or organic products.

Sunscreen is the best product you can use to protect your skin.

Do not believe everything you hear about skincare. Get the facts from reputable sources, not the local grapevine.

Chapter 14:
Ancient Beauty Rituals

There is a comfort in rituals, and rituals provide a framework for stability when you are trying to find answers.

Rituals help us to ground, concentrate, and calm the mind. Many sports players go through rituals before their big moments on the field or court; small movements and habits to calm and concentrate.

Deborah Norville, the longest-serving American TV anchor, won much acclaim during her career of more than two decades. Few people get two Emmy awards, work full time, stay happily married, and raise three children without a stable foundation. She survived a cancer scare and is the epitome of beauty and brains. How she does it, only she will know, but rituals give her stability in her busy New York life.

This chapter traces ancient beauty rituals practised over many centuries. Ancient though they may be, these rituals still resonate with modern-day skincare: baths for hygiene, moisturisers to protect the skin, perfume to celebrate life's flowers and spices, hair removal for smooth, sensual skin, and the ancient truth that health and beauty go hand in hand.

Medicine and Beauty Rituals Through the Ages

Beauty in early times was not a feminine issue. Beauty was part of medical practices, and the 21st century saw a partial return to the belief that health is a prerequisite for beauty. Modern experts recommend a healthy lifestyle as the first step in skincare and fighting the signs of ageing.

Ancient Medical and Cosmetic Books

For centuries, beauty was an essential part of medicine, and many ancient authors included beauty in their medical scripts:

- Galen, a Greek physician in the Roman empire, worried about beauty treatments interrupting medical emergencies. He gave precedence to medical treatments but was willing to make an exception for aristocrats wanting beauty treatments. He had recipes for balding heads and those desiring a different hair colour.

- Doctor Abu'al-Qasim Al Zahrawi, the Spanish pioneer of surgery in the Middle Ages, wrote Al Tasreef, a medical encyclopaedia of 30 volumes. It included skincare and cosmetic treatments.

- Ovid, the Roman poet quoted in Chapter 2, gave five recipes for facial lotions in one of his poems.

- The Persian physician, Avicenna, wrote The Canon of Medicine, a rule book used up to the 17th century. The Canon also included beauty advice.

- *De Ornatu Mulierum*, published early in the second century, listed 96 plant species. Monasteries were learning centres, and monks gathered information about plants and minerals for medical and cosmetic purposes.

- Doctor Sun Simiao's medical book, *Supplements to the Formulas of a Thousand Gold Worth*, was written during the Chinese Tang Dynasty and emphasised how closely related beauty and medicine were. It had a section on bath beans with a long list of ingredients: soybean powder (which contains isoflavones), herbs, and fragrances. For adventurous (or desperate) women, doctor Simiao suggests adding a pig pancreas and pig fat to combat the signs of ageing.

Ancient Medical and Cosmetic Practices

Ingredients From the Garden

The practice of homemade beauty treatments is a ritual; growing, harvesting, extracting the oil, grinding, and mixing followed the seasons. Archaeologists found 6,000-year-old remains of skincare and cosmetic rituals in Egypt, proving that the Egyptians used cosmetics not only for skincare and make-up but also as protection from the sun, insects, and other pests. They used what their gardens offered, and one can imagine the slave women collecting moringa tree leaves, castor beans, and sesame seeds, to which they added milk and honey. These rituals shaped the days of the lady of the house and the slaves who pampered her.

Ochre: Beauty and Medicine

Men and women in ancient Australia used ochre as decoration, wound treatment, and protection against the harsh climate and insect bites. Women painted only their faces, but the men covered their entire bodies with red ochre clay mixed with animal fats. They were proud warriors carrying spears and displaying their strength unashamedly.

Wilgi was war paint, medicine, and part of the ritual of life in the harsh Australian outback.

The Himba is a small tribe in northwest Namibia that uses *otjize*, a mixture of ochre and butterfat, to honour their land's soil. The red colour is a symbol of blood, life's essence. Like the Australian indigenous people, *otjize* is decorative but also protects against extreme weather conditions and insect bites.

However, Himba rituals also include intricate ochre headdresses. A Himba teenager starts planning her hair during puberty and builds on it for the rest of her life. *Otjize* rituals celebrate the seasons of womanhood: her readiness for marriage, her marital status, and the birth of her children.

Body treatments start with a smoke bath, after which ochre mixed with fat and fragrant herbs is rubbed into the body. Women sit together, talk, and massage *otjize* into each others' bodies. Through their ochre beauty care, they tell their individual stories against the backdrop of their traditions.

Bathing Rituals Across the Globe and Time

The history of public baths is as old as the human need for personal hygiene and care. Whether self-care and hygiene fall under the first of Maslow's needs (physiological) or the fourth (esteem) does not really matter. What matters is that humans go through rituals to feel better and to look good.

Over the centuries, many cultures used public baths for cleaning because people did not have bathrooms. But public baths were communal visiting places, much like the shopping malls in the 21st century. People went there to be cleaned but also to socialise. Even in modern society, having a long, hot bath, whether in a spa or your own bathroom, has a spiritual dimension: Be still and make time for yourself and those things in life that cannot be bought with money.

During the Roman and Byzantine eras, public bathing spread throughout the empire and arrived in Turkey during the 7th century. It was the centre of society, and people celebrated special events like weddings and the birth of a child at public baths.

A bathhouse usually had three rooms, including a hot steam room to get rid of the toxins. The rich lay on a central marble slab where attendants scrubbed them down. They then progressed to the second room for a long, hot bath. They were pampered with oils while cooling down and resting in the last room.

The poor washed each other's backs while enjoying the company of friends and neighbours.

A Brick Pool in the Indus Valley

In the early 1900s, archaeologists found one of the oldest public baths yet in the Indus Valley in present-day Pakistan. They excavated a relatively well-kept brick pool among the ruins.

A Bath Spirit in Russia

More to the east, in present-day Russia, Slavic myths tell about a bath (banya) spirit who would throw boiling water at a misbehaving bather. A strange ritual from the Russian Slavic ancestors has survived. Bathers hit themselves with birch twigs to open the pores and improve blood circulation. Traditionally, it also had a spiritual meaning – self-punishment and redemption.

A Spiritual Sweat Dome in Mexico

On the other side of the world, long before the Spaniards arrived in their sail ships in Mexico, the Aztecs believed steam promoted spiritual and physical health. Ancient Aztecs gathered in a dome-shaped sweat lodge built from volcanic rock. The dome shape symbolised a womb, a place of rebirth to replenish body and soul.

Attendees formed a circle around a pile of smouldering rocks. The spiritual leader poured water on the rocks every now and then, and steam filled the space. While their bodies were softened and pores opened to receive the blessings, the bathers sang and praised the spirits.

Sweat bathing was an intense spiritual experience, cleaning the body and strengthening character and morals.

Social Bathing and Mint Tea in Morocco

Hamman bathing is one of Africa's oldest beauty rituals. Many homes lacked bathrooms, and a weekly visit to the neighbourhood Hamman was necessary for personal hygiene. Equally important, the Hamman is a communal place to socialise. True to Islamic culture, women and men bathed separately; specific days were reserved for men and other days for women.

Moroccans are proud of their black or beldi soap, and every family has its own recipe. The base mixture usually is pureed olives and glycerin to which lavender, rose, or lemon oil might be added. One can also buy beldi at the market; soft but not runny. It is sold by the scoop in a plastic bag, or you can take your own bottle.

Often family members scrub each other's bodies, but an attendant will step in for a small fee. After the hot steam bath, women cool down, dress, and have a cup of mint tea with friends before returning to their chores back home. The weekly bathing is so much more than personal hygiene: It is a ritual of self-care, rest for body and soul, and socialising.

Natural Hot Springs in Japan

Japan has numerous hot springs because of its ever-present volcanic activities. When Buddhists arrived during the first century, public bathing in thermal pools became popular. Modern experts warn against the drying effect of extended hot baths, but Japanese women believe stress relief is vital for skin beauty. The hot baths open the pores while they exfoliate with sea salt, apply rice water for collagen formation, and finish with essential oils from flowers.

Milk and Jade in Korea

Korean public bathing is a daily affair, and everybody from grandparents to babies participates. Public baths are usually open day and night for a body scrub with milk and a jade massage for joint pain.

Milk Baths in Egypt

Who does not know of Elizabeth Taylor in a saffron-infused milk bath on the Nile capturing the attention of Richard Burton? Cleopatra bathed in donkey milk, and legend has it that 7,000 donkeys were needed to provide her with this luxury (Alex, 2016).

Lactic acid mildly exfoliates the skin and contains minerals and essential fatty acids. Saffron has numerous benefits for the skin. Cleopatra's extravagance was not the rule in Egypt, though. The wealthier people bathed at home because they had water channels running through their bathhouses. The poor bathed in the Nile using soap made from ash and clay.

Smoke Bridal Baths in Sudan

Sudanese *dukhan,* or smoke baths, are common among women to treat specific medical conditions and relax. Men taking smoke baths are frowned upon, but couples often enjoy a smoke bath together.

Sudanese brides follow a special ritual to prepare themselves for marriage. The bride, her body covered in oil, sits in a smoke bath fired by sweet-smelling acacia wood twice a week. She does not shower until the day of the marriage. The skin is soft and glowing when the smoky residue is eventually washed off.

Mud Bathing

People bathed in volcanic mud for centuries, as the ash contains several chemical substances, excellent for exfoliation and softening the skin. Mud's chemical components make it highly active: It detoxifies and relieves skin diseases, muscle pains, and general aches.

Mud hot spots are distributed across the globe. Romania's Lake Techirghiol is famous for its moor mud, containing sodium, chlorine, potassium, calcium, and sulphur. On the other side of the world, California's Napa Valley and Columbia also offer volcanic ash mud baths.

Mud is relatively hot, and people with chronic diseases should consult a doctor before taking mud therapy.

Salt Bathing in the Dead Sea

The Dead Sea is the lowest point on earth and, for many centuries, has been famous for hypersaline mud in which one can drift without care. No less than 21 minerals soothe the skin. The best known probably is Epson salts, renowned for its antiseptic and health benefits.

Besides skin benefits, Dead Sea salt and mud baths help with many medical conditions: psoriasis, asthma, and sinusitis. The air around the Dead Sea is virtually free of pollens, as no plant can grow in highly saline soil. Consequently, people with allergies find relief in its salt waters.

Hair Removal Rituals Across the Globe

Hair might be the most fickle feature in fashion: Some don't want it, others want curly, and still others desire straight hair. In the world of hair, there is indeed no dull moment.

Since the beginning of time, hair has played a vital role in personal care. Millions of years ago, humans had fur to protect them in the forests where they lived. As they moved and settled in open fields, they lost most of their body hair, as the hotter climate made it redundant. However, up until today, hair protects the scalp of humans.

Archaeological Evidence of Hair Removal

Cave pictures show hair removal rituals from many centuries ago, mostly women with long, braided locks. Their long braids were probably not shampooed and brushed as in modern times and must have been quite smelly. Interestingly, drawings of men show them without hair. Archaeologists guess the men, traditionally the hunters, did not want the aroma of unkept locks to forewarn their prey. Thus they shaved their heads. They also did not want to give the enemy something to grab and hold onto during a fight.

Archaeological records show that Oriental and Mediterranean women were already removing unwanted hair 4,000 years ago. In most ancient cultures, noble ladies removed all body hair, as hair was seen as uncivilised. Their wax consisted of a paste of arsenic sulphide, quicklime, and starch, which was left to dry on the skin and then ripped off.

An Egyptian medical book from 1500 B.C. gave a recipe for hair removal. Lotus leaves were burnt and the ashes mixed with grounded tortoiseshell and hippo fat.

Paintings and Writings

Paintings through the centuries tell a fascinating story of female beauty. Page through an art book, and you will see that goddesses and earthly women were always without body hair.

For many centuries, a high forehead was the epitome of beauty, and women removed about an inch of the hairline to raise the forehead. The preference for a high forehead continued for many centuries, and women used whatever they could to remove about an inch from the hairline.

It became the height of fashion during the reign of Elizabeth I during the 16th century. She removed her eyebrows as well. Some women stuck mouse skin for artificial brows higher up to extend the forehead. More affluent women slowed down regrowth with walnut oil, but the ordinary women had to make do with a mixture of cat faeces and vinegar (Mackay, 1989). The latter proves that not all rituals were necessarily pleasant.

Middle Eastern Halawa, or Sugaring

Halawa, or sugaring, is still a popular hair removal method in the Middle East. Sugaring is a century-old method to remove hair and was used in ancient Egypt. Honey was initially used, but in modern salons, sugar is mixed with lemon juice and left to dry on the body.

As the ingredients are natural, the risk of allergies is lower. Also, the sugar paste does not settle on the skin but around the hairs. When ripped off, the hair is removed without hurting the skin. It is thus not the same as waxing with a resin.

In North Africa, sugaring is a monthly ritual where women gather and sugar each other. These meetings are far more than beauty treatments: It is the place to talk, share, relax, and encourage each other through difficult times.

From Sea Shells to Gillette

The razor's forerunner was probably a sharp knife-like object made from stone or shells. Ancient Egyptian men and women had razors made from flint and bronze to remove facial and body hair. In the late 18th century, a French barber designed a razor with a wooden handle. According to reports from that era, it was safer and caused fewer wounds.

The name Gillette is synonymous with razors, and many teenage girls 'borrowed' their father's Gillette on the sly. Gillette, an American businessman, not only designed the first safety razor but also patented the first disposable razor.

In the early 20th century, fashion moved from the prudish Victorian age to modernism. Sleeveless dresses became fashionable, and women started shaving their armpits. Once again, Gillette stepped in and designed the first razor just for women. And, as the saying goes, the rest is history.

Electrolysis is a modern development, and many women threw out their razors forever. You might not think of electrolysis as a relaxing skincare ritual. For women with unwanted hair, it is a ritual of hope to be savoured bit by bit during each treatment. Modern electrolysis has roots in medical research in treating ingrowing eyelashes, further evidence of how closely related the cosmetic and medical fields are. Its story develops in the next chapter.

Perfume Rituals in the Great Empty Quarter

Perfumes were traditionally not applied to the skin but taken orally as medicine. They were homemade remedies made from the orchard's flowers and fruits. In the 19th century, perfume as we know it today became a status symbol for the wealthy, made with a single 'note', as the perfumiers call it.

But the actual value of perfume lies in the preceding ritual of cleaning the body and donning fresh clothes. The final step of this self-care ritual is a dash of perfume, which says: I have time for me. I honour myself and my body. I celebrate life's abundance with this perfume.

Ancient Perfumes

The oldest cultures in the world used perfume: Chinese, Roman, Arabic, Egypt, Cyprus, and the earliest inhabitants of the Indus Valley. Initially, perfumes were used to honour the gods, send prayers to heaven, purify the dead, and as medication. Less spiritual and more practical was the use of perfume to camouflage the stank of urine and faeces in the streets of Rome.

In 16th-century England, all public places were sprinkled with perfumes, and ladies travelled in their coaches with small perfume bottles to keep the stank of the masses at bay.

Archaeologists found remnants of incense in Kyphi, an ancient Egyptian perfume. A written record exists of Hungary Water, made for the queen of Hungary in 1370 (Kristic, 2021). Perfume history and perfume rituals have a rich history and deserve a book of their own.

Let's look at one of the most unlikely areas to produce the ingredients for perfumes, the Great Empty Quarter and the world's most feared desert.

Perfumes of Arabia

The history of Arabian perfumery dates back to the 6th century and its religious origins. Perfume forms an integral part of Arabian religious life. Roughly translated and with sincere respect, the Prophet Muhammad advised the following ritual: taking a bath on Friday is compulsory for every male, cleaning the teeth with Miswak, and using perfume if available. Miswak is a twig that, when chewed, frays and acts as a brush.

Middle-Eastern perfumes have dark undertones, reminiscent of the harsh environment from where they originate. Through the centuries, Arabians used the sparse gifts of their desert vegetation for perfume making, and Bedouins still harvest frankincense and myrrh as their ancestors did many centuries ago.

Frankincense and myrrh are indigenous to the southeast of the Arabian Peninsula and have been known since Biblical times when the three wise men brought them to the baby Jesus as gifts. Harvesting myrrh and frankincense has changed little over the centuries and is deeply embedded in desert life.

Small incisions of about two inches are made in the tree's bark. The tree 'cries' and secretes a milky liquid that hardens into 'tears'. The harvester checks for the tears to become opaque or silvery, sometimes up to five times. In the olden days, the silver tears were sold to passing merchant caravans. Nowadays, they are delivered directly to the perfumery.

Oman is centrally situated on the ancient marine silk route. The flavours, fashions, and fetishes of sailors from all over the world enriched their perfume culture: sandalwood and Oudh from India, cedars from Lebanon, and oak moss from the forests of Europe. Patchouli leaves (related to mint) come from Sri Lanka, and their masculine tone is suitable for men's perfumes.

The names of the flowers alone remind one of a spring garden: jasmine, lily of the valley, violets, peach blossoms, and the most famous, roses. About two hours' drive from Muscat is Jabal al Akhder, a mountain town, even today only accessible by four-wheel-drive vehicles. For centuries, rose pickers have gathered and dried the small pink buds during April to make rose oil and rose water.

Arabian perfume also contains plum and fig flavours and the spicey aroma of vanilla, cardamom, and cinnamon.

Surrounded by no less than five seas (The Red Sea, Arabian Sea, Gulf of Aden, Gulf of Oman, and the Persian Gulf), the Arabians also use the sea's treasures. Ambergris is a solid, dull grey substance produced in the digestive system of sperm whales and collected from beaches far and wide. It has a peculiarly sweet, earthy odour and is a fixative in perfume.

Skin Protection Across the Globe and the Centuries

Taking care of oneself is as old as human history. The world's most prominent religions agree on the importance of skincare and health: The Psalmist in the Christian and Jewish Bible speaks about the blessing of oil for the skin. The Prophet believed in proactively caring for the skin and warned about sun avoidance.

Mediaeval and Renaissance Women

From archaeological and written sources, we know that women in mediaeval times valued smooth, white skin and used homemade products for skincare. They used cucumber juice with a shot of vinegar to clean, boiled oats in vinegar to treat acne, and soaked bread in rose water to relieve puffy eyes.

Also, moisturisers were made from their garden and farming produce. They slowly melted fats from their animals over low heat until the proteins solidified and the water evaporated. They then filtered the fat and added herbs and plant extracts from the garden: aloe vera, rosemary, flowers, and seed oil.

From Leeches to Lead – Dying for Beauty?

White skin with red cheeks was the ultimate look in mediaeval times. The early Egyptians used pigments from oils and herbs to colour their cheeks and lips, but Roman women used anything from animal urine, poultry poop, sulphur, white lead, egg whites, and vinegar to lighten the skin. These ointments were often so strong that they burnt the skin.

To look pale, they put leeches on the ears and cheeks to suck the blood from their faces. They covered wounds with small star-shaped fabrics, which doubled as decoration.

The desire for white skin took a frightening turn: Women used red lead for rosy cheeks. The effect on health was potentially horrendous, but the trend continued for centuries.

Today we know lead dehydrates the skin and reduces elasticity. It can cause kidney problems, damage to the nervous system, and skin lesions.

The use of toxins in make-up continued right up to the Victorian period. Advertisements of the era offered 'safe' arsenic soap, ammonia, opium, and mercury. Statistics on arsenic poisoning in the Victorian era are not available, as it was only later realised how toxic arsenic was. They also used silver, mercury, and chalk to colour their faces.

Professor Fiona McNeill of Canada researched recipes containing lead from the 16th to the 19th century with exciting results even for today's women. They found that white lead make-up gave the skin a subtle whiteness, not as mask-like as it usually is portrayed in film reproductions (McNeill, 2022).

Also, lead is poisonous when inhaled or eaten, but fortunately, the skin does not readily absorb it. However, Elizabeth I used a highly toxic recipe of lead mixed with vinegar. It is absorbed by the skin and can cause deadly lead poisoning.

Eyebrowless Elizabethan England

Nonetheless, the eyebrowless Queen Elizabeth I of England, with her red hair and milkwhite skin, became the symbol of beauty in the late 16th century.

Hygiene was highly rated, and ladies bathed in 'Soloman's Water'. It contained high mercury concentrations and, depending on the concentration, could remove the upper layer, leaving the skin raw and infected.

Fashionable ladies finally realised that rotting teeth were gruesome and made toothpaste from honey, crushed bones, and fruit peel.

Mediterranean and Middle Eastern Women Used Nature's Gifts

Mediterranean cuisine is unthinkable without olive oil, and ancient Greeks used olive oil as the base for most skincare products. They added fresh garden ingredients like berries, honey, milk, and yoghurt to exfoliate and moisturise the skin.

The Middle East is a desert with limited botanical resources to make skincare products. Women in Egypt and Europe had lavender, roses, jasmine, and violets. Arabian women ingeniously used what they could find in the desert: camel milk, frankincense, saffron, and the extremely bitter myrrh, currently buzzwords in western beauty circles.

Bedouin women believed for centuries what modern chemists only recently discovered. Myrrh prevents tissue degeneration and, apart from medical properties, has a rejuvenating effect on the skin. Mixed with animal fat, it was an excellent moisturiser for dry, flaky skin and removed toxins, thus promoting tissue repair.

The Bedouins believed camel milk was an aphrodisiac, as camels could go up to 14 days without drinking water. They never used the milk on the first night after a period without water, as they believed the milk was poisonous.

Another favourite ingredient was sandalwood oil extracted from the wood itself. A small piece of wood was tirelessly ground on a stone and mixed with a dash of any other oil. Today a touch of vaseline helps the slow grinding process.

Minute pinches of saffron enriched the woody-smelling sandalwood oil.

Ayurveda in India

Already 5000 years ago, Sanskrit scripts emphasised a holistic approach to health. Later texts, called Brhattrayi, are the foundation of Ayurveda as it is still practised today. The Sanskrit word *Ayur* means life, and *Veda* means science or knowledge.

Ayurveda believes that imbalance and stress cause disease and that one can regain balance through natural processes and herbal remedies. Treatment aims to remove the impurities in the body, supplemented by herbal therapies and a special diet. However, Ayurveda strongly believes that the spirit must heal through meditation, yoga, and massage.

Ayurvedic skincare addresses stress and pollution. Similar to the skin types discussed in Chapter 2, Ayurveda classifies the skin in categories of *doshas*:

Vata – dry, cracked, and ages quickly

Pitta – fair, thin, sensitive, acne-prone, freckled, moles, and ages moderately fast

Kapha – normal or oily, clear, smooth, and does not age so quickly

Each woman has a primary *dosha*, but it can be influenced by environmental factors such as pollution, sun damage, and lifestyle habits. Ayurvedic products require a routine of topical products and massages. It is a slow physical and spiritual purification process that helps you see your life through a holistic lens for greater perspective and peace. Ayurvedic treatment over an extended period encompasses more than physical healing; it strives for spiritual healing and growth.

The success of the Ayurvedic holistic approach and herbal treatments is globally appreciated, and Ayurvedic treatments are available in every country. The Association of Ayurvedic Professionals has coordinated the practices in the United Kingdom since 2018. Ayurvedic products are regulated as dietary supplements in the United States, and ayurvedic schools must be licensed.

Far East

In the Far East, women used safflower seeds, rice powder, imported sesame seed oil, jasmine, rose water, and spices such as cloves to beautify themselves. During the Tang dynasty, Chinese women shaped their eyebrows like silkworms, celebrating the sericulture that made their country rich and famous. By replicating the curve of a silkworm on their faces, they declared themselves proudly part of the hustle and bustle of the silkworm industry.

Japanese women used rice water, green tea, and turmeric as moisturisers. They used water saved from rice cooking for its starch, vitamins, and proteins. Geishas had to keep their skin young and supple to please their clients and avoided dehydrated, harsh soaps. They used creams to clean the face and camellia oil as a luxurious skin treatment.

Quick Reminder

Through centuries, men and women have cared for their appearances. Where nothing else was available, they made their own oils and treatments.

The beauty and medical worlds have overlapped since mediaeval times, and a healthy lifestyle is a prerequisite for good skin.

The rituals surrounding beauty enrich the spirit as much as it enhances the appearance.

The concept of what is beautiful differs from age to age, but a well-kept woman never goes out of fashion.

Chapter 15:
Skincare and Modern History

Beauty on duty has a duty to beauty.

During the Second World War, an advertisement for Victory red lipstick illustrates how deeply entrenched the beauty industry was in the stark realities of the war. Today many people will object to the 'Beauty is Duty' slogan, but at the time, it boosted morale, according to Pat Spicer, a young dressmaker during the war. 'There was so much poverty and danger, we craved glamour and escapism', she reflected in *The Daily Mirror* (Thompson, 2021).

Every era's beauty practices reflect the traditions and culture of its society. Women were energised by and reacted to their environment in their expression of skin – and beauty care. These practices and trends tell us about a society and reveal the values, religious norms, and attitudes behind its traditions and culture.

Beauty rituals and trends of the early times are discussed in the previous chapter. This chapter gives an overview of the last hundred years.

Beauty Developments During the Past Century

The Late 19th Century

The Industrial Revolution from the 1850s onward was a turning point in Europe's modern history. Not surprisingly, skincare and beauty perceptions of the time followed the economic trends. Women benefitted from education opportunities, and with new-found knowledge, they soon realised that health is an essential aspect of beauty. A new sense of healthy living developed, and exercise and hygiene became increasingly important.

Dangerous metals were no longer used, and manufacturers became more aware of the health properties of beauty products' ingredients.

Unfortunately, the preference for lighter skin continued up to the 1960s. Light skin was a sign of privilege, a necessity to distinguish society ladies from the working classes. Working-class women had to work in the sun and, therefore, had darker skin. Fashionistas used zinc oxide, lemon juice, honey, egg yolks, and oatmeal paste to bleach and moisturise the skin.

Straight hair was for long the trend, and the larger-than-life Madame C. J. Walker took on the curls of her African descent. She became the first African-American millionaire by selling her straightening devices and products. She had lost most of her hair because of a scalp disease and developed a scalp preparation and iron combs. An entrepreneur at heart, her success propelled her into developing other hair products for African-American women. Selling from home to home, she supported herself and her daughter. Her business grew, and she later opened a beauty school and a factory. And the rest, as the saying goes, is history.

Industrialisation and Vaseline

The beauty industry as an economic force is relatively young: It only emerged as an independent business sector in the 19th century (Silverthorne, 2010). Industrialisation and the petroleum industry changed the world and also beauty care forever. Vaseline is the single most enduring byproduct of the petrochemical industry. More than a century and a half after Robert Chesebrough, a New York pharmacist, started his experiments, Vaseline is still a stalwart for dry and damaged skin.

As beauty and skincare developed, chemists refined Vaseline into a non-greasy substance still used in most modern skincare products. It contains mineral oil known as paraffin wax, a humectant that attracts and binds with moisture to prevent dehydration.

The First World War

The First World War further changed the beauty landscape drastically. With the men fighting, women had to drive taxis and work in factories, and for the first time, scores of women earned their own income. Women loved their emancipation, having their own money, and spending some of it on themselves.

Where Egypt, the Far, and the Middle East were antiquity's beauty hotspots, Europe and America became the epicentre of the booming cosmetic business. The beauty industry in the

West flourished. Beauty salons developed, from secretive back rooms suspected of being brothels to the luxurious, highly hygienic spas and studios of modern times.

European and American beauty legends became the topic of many books, plays, and movies. Greta Garbo, her looks reflecting strength and character, was the symbol of beauty in the earlier part of the 20th century.

As women started wearing light, sleeveless summer dresses, unwanted hair became an issue. Soon, shaving seemed not good enough, and doctors looked for more permanent solutions. In the 1920s, x-rays were considered very effective in removing unwanted hair. A decade later, the deadly effect of radiation became apparent, and many women died of cancer.

Although skincare and health became the norm, society still frowned upon make-up. It was seen as 'fast' and was associated with loose women. Initially, women used cosmetics sparingly and hoped it would be seen as natural colouring. Working class women were the first to daringly apply red lipstick and rouge. Society ladies gossiped but gradually followed the trend.

Early 20th Century Beauty Legends

Some of the big names in the beauty world originated from that time: Coty, Helena Rubenstein, Elizabeth Arden, Vinolia, and Pears. Advertisements during the war encouraged women to keep up their appearances: 'The inconveniences of war need not interfere with a beauty regime' (Gosling, 2013).

Also, in the early 20th century, the women's rights movement took off, and red lipstick accidentally became the symbol of emancipation. In 1912, protesting suffragettes walked past the office of Elizabeth Arden, a women's rights advocate in her own right. Arden handed out red lipsticks to show her support, inadvertently causing 15,000 women with red lips to take on the New York patriarchal society.

In Europe, ordinary women gained access to perfume which was previously mostly the prerogative of the aristocracy. Until the turn of the 20th century, perfume was sold in medicine bottles. One man, the flamboyant Francois Coty, appointed a glass designer for his elegant perfume bottles, and ever since, women love their bit of luxury in a pretty bottle.

According to legend, Francois Coty deliberately smashed a bottle of La Rose Jacqueminot in the upmarket store Grands Magasins du Louvre in Paris. This perfume was made from a hybrid rose, and its fragrance overwhelmed the women shoppers. Coty got his first order and an entire display window to advertise his perfume.

Coty did not stop in Europe. He sent his mother-in-law to America, making Coty a household name in perfumes, skincare, and make-up.

Two other legends in the beauty industry, Helena Rubenstein and Elizabeth Arden, had a life-long competition to be the best in the beauty industry. Their feud carried on for nearly 50 years. *Warpaint*, a book and later a musical, is based on their story of rivalry.

The Great Depression and Hollywood

The 1930s saw a global collapse of the economy, and even more, women started working outside the home. At the same time, Hollywood exploded, and women copied the styles of the great actresses of the time, wearing make-up defiantly. Make-up finally made it onto every dressing table as women grew confident to live according to their standards, not those of puritan society.

The Second World War

As the Second World War developed, women had to step into men's positions again in factories, on the streets, and on the farms. Dressed in overalls, they wanted to keep their femininity, and red lipstick became fashionable again. Despite the horror of war, women still wanted to look good. As women replaced men in the workforce, red lipstick grew in popularity.

In the U.K., the prime minister Winston Churchill encouraged women to stay stylish and keep up appearances. Many companies handed out red lipstick to boost the morale of their women workers.

During the war, manufacturers needed nylon for parachutes, aeroplane cords, and ropes, and a shortage of nylon stockings forced women to shave their legs. Back in the 1940s, no decent lady could leave her house without stockings.

Hitler and Lipstick

Interestingly, red lipstick once again symbolised patriotism, especially as Hitler strongly disapproved of make-up. He believed German women of Aryan descent did not need any make-up and recommended that they also did not wear jewellery, perfume, fur, or trousers. Hitler, a vegetarian, especially disliked lipstick, as it contained animal fats. Women were warned not to wear lipstick or have painted nails in Hitler's vicinity.

Allied women might not have fought actively in the trenches of Europe, but they proudly wore perfume and red lipstick in defiance of Nazism. A made-up look was regarded as a patriotic sign, a woman doing her bit to keep the morale high in the terrible war times. It oozed confidence and showed their patriotism.

Montezuma and Victory Lipsticks

In the United States, the government asked Elizabeth Arden to create a special red lipstick for women who joined the army, Montezuma Red. The name personified strength as it was derived from *Angry Like a Lord,* the name of the last independent ruler of the Aztec leader, Motecuhzoma or Moctezuma (Cartwright, 2013). Civilian ladies got their shade of red, defiantly called Victory Red.

With blond hair, red lips, good legs, and sensuality, Marilyn Monroe was the epitome of what the 20th-century man saw as beautiful. Many women might have objected, but 50 years later, Andy Warhol's poster of Marilyn still decorates the interiors of private homes and public spaces.

The World Becomes a Global Village

During the second half of the 20th century, and based on the immense technological developments, more and more people knew what was happening at any place, any time, anywhere on the planet. With this newfound freedom came a strong sense of independence. Women expressed themselves through make-up and fashion – sometimes reinterpreting the past and other times, creating new trends.

Beauty was a way to express anger and protest against moral issues such as animal cruelty, gender violence, child labour, racial disparities, and climate change.

Make-Up Through the Decades

The 1960s saw heavy eyeliner, pale lips, and mini dresses. Women in the 1970s loved tie dye, peasant blouses, and bell bottoms. And who will ever forget the 1980s with its big hair? In the 1990s, women and men in tight shirts and platform shoes braved the streets to show off their studded accessories. The 2000s saw women in shorts and designer bags. Since then, everything goes army boots with a light summer dress; hats and heels and faux leather in protest against animal cruelty.

21st Century

The beauty industry is enormous and worth billions of dollars. It is a tough business, and the movie *The Devil Wears Prada* with Meryl Streep and Anne Hathaway gave us a glimpse into the lonely world of glitter and glamour.

Furthermore, the 21st-century consumer increasingly disregards products based on gender. Fluidity in skincare is once again accepted as normal, as it had been many centuries ago in mediaeval times. People of all genders want skincare products to maintain skin quality and address their problems, believing that caring for oneself is a fundamental human privilege.

Cosmeceutical products

No wonder cosmeceutical products with medical and cosmetic properties make up a significant portion of the present beauty market. The word 'cosmeceutical' is still not clearly defined. Some see it as a cross between medical and cosmetic research, and Japan calls it quasi-drugs. The term was first used in 1984 by Dr Albert Kligman of the University of Pennsylvania. He researched the anti-ageing effects of tretinoin. It inspired him to define cosmeceutical products as having pharmaceutical and cosmetic benefits (Pandey, 2021).

The precise definition of cosmeceutical products differs from country to country. Still, it is generally accepted that the following products are cosmeceuticals: sunscreen, skin lightening and depigmentation, moisturisers, anti-ageing, scar-reducers, hair strengtheners, alpha-hydroxy acids, topical retinol (vitamin C), and antioxidants.

Light Emitting Diodes

Technological developments in various industries also benefitted the beauty industry. LED light therapy is discussed in Chapter 9, but its history deserves special mention. NASA first used it in the 1990s when astronauts experimented with different light colours to grow veggies in space (Arné, n.d.).

Magic and Smart Mirrors

The humble make-up mirror has wholly entered the 21st century, and smart mirrors now have a built-in skin analyser. It scans your face and recommends appropriate skincare products. Smart mirrors go further and suggest the correct shades for your make-up products. Some companies call it a personal dermatologist (Saini, 2020).

The smart mirror can never replace professional advice, especially not if you have serious concerns about your skin. A dermatologist will treat the symptoms and address the condition's causes, something the smart mirror can't do. You can learn more about artificial intelligence in skincare in Chapter 16.

Science and Beauty Meet in Electrolysis

Electrolysis developed independently from skincare and cosmetics, as it started in the surgeries of doctors confronted with the medical problem of ingrown eyelashes. In the medical world, trichiasis poses an uncomfortable and painful problem. A tiny object such as an eyelash can have devastating results when it grows inward and irritates the cornea.

In 1800, William Nicholson discovered electrolysis to separate water into hydrogen and oxygen. Electrolysis is a technique that uses an electric current to create a chemical reaction.

Three decades later, in 1834, Michale Faraday's research added a new theory to electrolysis called electrochemistry. He published his findings in a paper that has become known as 'Faraday's Two Laws of Electrolysis'. However, it took another four decades for electrolysis to be used for ingrown eyelashes.

Doctors experimented with chemical solutions to stop regrowth with varying degrees of success. In the middle of the 19th century, doctors in North America inserted a needle dipped in sulfuric acid into the hair follicle. They then injected carbolic acid into the bulb and twisted the needle. It stopped hair growth permanently but, understandably, was an intensely painful process that often left ugly scars.

American Civil War

Fast-forward to the end of the 19th century and the American Civil War. The ophthalmologist Dr Charles Michel began developing a less frightening process in 1869. A few years later, in 1875, he took the treatment to new levels. He permanently removed an ingrown eyelash by inserting a surgical needle into the hair follicle. The needle was attached to a dry cell. He then applied a current and took the hair out with tweezers. It was less painful and 100% successful, as the hair did not grow again.

In 1877, dermatologist Willam Hardaway used this new method for the first time as a cosmetic treatment. He and a colleague removed the unseemly beard from a 'thoroughly feminine in character and physique, nicely plumb and robustly healthy' 22-year-old. Strand by strand, they worked, and after 350 treatments, all beard hairs were removed (Permanence, n.d.).

Unfortunately, it is not documented what happened to the thoroughly feminine lady. However, judging by many women whose lives have since dramatically improved through electrolysis, she must have spent the rest of her days a happy woman.

Early 20th Century

During the next decade, chemical and thermal hair removal techniques developed side by side. In 1916, Professor Paul M Kree of New York first used the galvanic method, which chemically destroyed the hair follicle. He developed the technique into a six-needle method. His research and practice form the basis of the current galvanic method used globally. The galvanic method uses caustic lye to destroy regrowth.

On the other side of the world, in Lyon, France, Dr Henri Bordier developed what is today known as thermolysis. It is also called short-wave diathermy, which means 'to heat'. High-frequency energy waves heat the natural substances in the hair follicle (Electrolysis Beauty Lounge, n.d.).

At the end of World War II, Henri E St Pierre, in cooperation with the American engineer Arthur Hinkel, patented a device that combined galvanic and thermolysis techniques. Hinkel, who worked at the medical division of General Electric, met St Pierre in 1930. Still, it took more than a decade to develop and launch the concept of electrolysis to remove unwanted hair in 1948. The cooperation between these two men led to the blend method. The blend method's speed falls between that of galvanic and thermolysis.

The blend method is still the most successful and frequently used for unwanted facial and body hair (Electrolysis Beauty Lounge, n.d.). There are many other treatments and fashion trends to remove unwanted hair. Many offer a quick fix, but to this day – and underwritten by most governments – electrolysis is the only permanent hair removal method.

Black Beauty in the 20th Century

For centuries, white skin was treasured, and women took extreme measures to lighten their skin.

As far back as 1890, some communities in the United States organised beauty contests for black women. The black press picked up on this trend and published pictures of black women. However, even these joyful events were overshadowed by a preference for lighter complexions (Craig, 2017).

Until the mid-20th century, the mainstream media nearly exclusively covered white beauty and skincare. The 20th century saw a slow but steady awareness of black beauty and products aimed at people with dark skin.

With technological development and increased economic and educational opportunities for black women, the Black is Beautiful movement grew. The 1960s became a watershed decade in the black beauty industry. Similar to the world wars, beauty was intensely politicised. Up to that stage, the beauty industry focused on getting the skin lighter and the hair straighter, while being as thin as a matchstick.

Black is Beautiful rejected the century-old, narrow perception based on white skin and straight hair as the ultimate in beauty. Black women proudly displayed their ethnic hair, and various styles developed to celebrate its unique texture.

Unfortunately, centuries of prejudice cannot be wiped out in a few decades, and many black women still bleached their skin and straightened their hair. The preference for straight hair became one of the most contentious issues in the Black is Beautiful movement of the mid-20th century.

Several black women writers reported that beauty perceptions are deeply rooted in and defined by cultural prejudices. Other writers warned that the Black is Beautiful movement would be meaningless if women did not change their perceptions of their unique ethnic beauty.

Africa is densely populated, and the beauty industry has grown astonishingly over the last decade. Young women make up the most significant portion of the African beauty market. Therefore, it is not surprising that cosmetics make up the largest portion of the African beauty industry.

At the height of the global pandemic in 2021, the African beauty industry was worth multi-billions of dollars and is still growing. The epicentre of the growth in Nigeria and women in this densely populated but previously neglected continent are finally getting access to beauty and skincare (The Guardian, 2021).

The Global Pandemic and the Beauty Industry

The 21st century saw a growing concern about the environment and the sustainability of resources. When the global pandemic struck the world early in 2020, there was already a general perception that beauty should be more socially and environmentally responsible. The globally enforced, paired-down lifestyle enhanced this trend during the COVID-19 pandemic.

The COVID pandemic restricted many women to their homes and forced them to take their beauty care into their own hands. In pre-COVID times, women relied on outside advice, such as the beauty department at their local shop. Others bought products suggested by a beautician, but the situation changed drastically.

Millions of women turned to the internet to get advice and buy beauty items. Women bought less make-up and more skincare products because they had to stay home. Also, it seems like the extra me-time inspired women to become more informed about the products and their ingredients. COVID-19 made everybody extra health conscious, and this attitude is also reflected in the beauty market trends.

Sales show that women care about skin bacteria, pollution, and possible infections. They want products that take care of their skin and do not negatively impact the environment. People increasingly care about wasteful packaging, child labour, and sustainable ingredients.

As women spend long hours in front of their screens, scientists warned that digital blue light could damage the eyes and the skin. Online searchers for products to address this went sky-high. But what is blue light, and why, if at all, is it bad?

Blue light on our screens comes from light-emitting fluorescent light and can cause eye strain. Research on the effects of blue light is still confusing, but consumers can use screen protectors to filter out blue light.

Retailers did not only change their marketing strategies to direct online sales, but social networks now provide videos and assistance with every beauty and skincare aspect. Several beauty brands launched major online programmes; wherever the internet is, women now have access to the latest trends and techniques. Box subscriptions skyrocketed and became a significant segment of the beauty trade.

Beauty and hair salons also jumped on the internet wagon, and online bookings became the most effortless way to make an appointment. Furthermore, the client has the opportunity to complete an online form before their appointment, considerably cutting short admin and waiting time.

The pandemic changed not only how women shopped but once again proved that beauty is a major socio-economic and political weapon to address injustices and global issues. On the surface, beauty seems vain and superficial. Still, beauty and skincare are much more: It is not only the way a woman expresses her individuality but also an illustration of her values and a statement on how she views the world and its inhabitants.

Quick Reminder

Beauty and skincare have been highly politicised during the past century.

European and American women wore make-up, especially red lipstick, to keep their morale high during the world wars.

Special red lipsticks were launched in the United States during the Second World War. Military women wore Montezuma and civilian ladies Victory Red in defiance of Nazism and Hitler's dislike for make-up.

The 20th century saw the development of cosmeceutical skincare products meant to beautify and treat the skin simultaneously.

Consumers in the 21st century are acutely concerned about the environment and sustainability of resources; consequently, they hold manufacturers responsible for keeping the beauty industry clean and green.

Electrolysis is an example of how science and beauty combined to help women struggling with unwanted hair.

After centuries of neglect, the movement Black is Beautiful flourished during the last decades and is still growing, emphasising that women of all ethnic groups are uniquely beautiful.

The COVID-19 pandemic changed how women buy. Online shopping and consultation on skincare and cosmetics have become the norm.

Chapter 16:
The Future of Skincare

It is not faith in technology. It is faith in people.

The late Steve Jobs, the co-founder of Apple, believed technology should always be about people. This chapter speaks about the future of skincare, cosmetics, and plastic surgery, a future where women will have access to personalised products made from sustainable resources that are responsibly manufactured.

Modern women are more informed and will no longer be satisfied with meaningless marketing terms. They want published evidence on safety trials and sustainable ingredients.

The beauty industry is dynamic and has expanded to Asia and Africa. The following economic and personal trends are predicted for the beauty industry:

- The South Korean beauty market will grow significantly over the next five years.

- Asia and the South Pacific Islands will become the biggest market for skincare products.

- Africa's beauty industry will grow faster than the global average, especially the cosmetic market because young women comprise a large portion of the population.

- The online skincare market will keep growing.

- Artificial intelligence will play a significant role in skincare analysis, treatment options, and cosmetic sales.

- Consumers will increasingly buy skincare products, and make-up sales will decrease slightly.

- Consumers will increasingly insist on eco-friendly products that do not impact the environment negatively.

Biocosmetics

Global warming, floods, unprecedented heat waves, and other natural disasters contributed to consumer awareness of green and sustainable beauty products. Consequently, manufacturers strive to replace fossil-based with bio-based ingredients, which is a challenging and expensive process.

Biocosmetics are entirely made of natural extracts from plants, animals, insects, enzymes, and microbes (organisms too small to see with the human eye). Furthermore, chemicals are not allowed during production. It is a tall order, as many countries don't yet have legislation or the financial means to manage organic production.

Also, biocosmetics must be preservative-free, considerably shortening the product's shelf life. No animal testing is tolerated. And of utmost importance, packaging must be compostable.

Nonetheless, the sustainable and natural green products market is growing, as consumers increasingly resist skincare products made with fossil-based ingredients. Popular ingredients include extracts from coconut, ginger root, cactus, prickly pears, rumex (perennial herbs), willow bark, apricot kernels, and safflower seeds.

Producing entirely organic products free from chemicals is challenging, and production is expensive. Furthermore, agriculture is a seasonal industry, and shortages during the off-season pose problems. Researchers thus explore many other options.

The world's oceans offer several bio-active ingredients such as marine bacteria, micro-algae and halophytes (plants with a high salt tolerance). But this industry also has many safety issues, as marine pollution is a major and global problem.

Food-based ingredients such as minerals, vitamins, lipids, proteins, and carbohydrates are excellent antioxidants and lend themselves to biocosmetic production. Peptides are the buzzword in this field, and researchers distinguish between several types of peptides: signal peptides, carrier peptides, or neurotransmitter inhibiting peptides. Peptides assist in skin permeation and stabilising the active ingredients.

Unfortunately, few skincare products with marine- and food-based biocosmetics are market-ready yet. More research on their safety is necessary.

An exciting development is the use of food waste in the biocosmetic industry. The food industry generates an enormous amount of waste. Researchers experiment with extractions from vegetable peels, orange peel, groundnut oil cake, ashes, clays, seeds, sugarcane, broccoli stalks, leaves, roots, husks, coffee grounds, and molasses. However, the risk of toxicity is high, and more testing is necessary before these extractions will be generally used in skincare products.

Global standards and regulations are adapted to make way for biocosmetics to replace fossil-based products. Total transparency is necessary, which poses a challenge given the size of the beauty industry. The following certifications for biocosmetics already exist: Ecocert (France), Cosmébio (Canada), USDA (United States), and BDIH (Germany).

Biocosmetics and Artificial Intelligence

Several leading companies use artificial intelligence in the development of biocosmetics. Artificial intelligence predicts how active molecules in bioproducts will react to the millions of natural microbial species (bacteria, yeast, fungi, viruses) on human skin. It is generally accepted that disturbances in the human skin's natural microbes contribute to many common skin conditions.

It is therefore vital that cosmeceutical products do not disturb the microbes on the skin. Artificial intelligence can select the appropriate bioactive ingredient and formulas to maintain the skin's microbes. It is used in face-mapping, identifying skin problems, and developing bioproducts to address these issues.

Artificial Intelligence and Metaverse in Skincare

Artificial Intelligence (AI) in skincare is a reality and will soon become a major diagnostic tool. The global COVID-19 pandemic forced manufacturers and retailers to enable consumers to self-analyse their skin type and identify its problems in the comfort of their own homes. Furthermore, consumers will have immediate access to online products and treatments.

Research has shown that 21st-century women are knowledgeable about their skincare products and demand reliable information on skincare ingredients and how they can improve skin quality. Moreover, they are willing to pay for scientifically backed products targeted at their individual needs.

Personalised Digital Skincare

Although technology seems cold and inhuman, artificial intelligence in skincare aims to do the opposite: personalised skincare for the 21st-century woman who is no longer satisfied with a moisturiser designed for a broad user category. The modern woman wants a product intended for her and is digitally savvy to manage analytical tools in the 'metaverse', as the virtual reality space is called.

A woman can now sit at her dressing table with her phone and identify a specific skin issue within seconds. This technology is growing and will provide exciting opportunities for consumers over the next few years. It will increasingly enable the consumer to address her skin issues with online treatments or get professional help.

Digital skincare technology already identifies and recommends products for several skin conditions: spots, texture, dark circles, oiliness, acne, droopy lower and upper eyelids, radiance, wrinkles, bags under the eyes, moisture levels, redness, firmness, and pores. This technology is expected to grow and branch out to other personal and healthcare fields.

So how does artificial intelligence work? With all make-up removed, hair tied back, and without glasses, the consumer sits in a well-lit area and looks straight into the phone's camera. Within seconds they receive a report with a summary of face shape, skin tone, eyelid form, eye colour, eyebrow shape and density, lip shape and colour, nose width and length, cheekbones, and hair colour.

A typical report might look like this: round face, softly angled brows, double-lid eyes, flat cheekbones, heavy underlip. Digital technology will allow you to try several products and techniques to enhance the features. You can try different products to reshape the face outline, enhance the cheekbones, camouflage the chin shape or length, and highlight the jawline.

If you wish to go beyond skincare, you can have your features analysed to determine your personality: Are you an extrovert? An agreeable, conscientious person who is open to new experiences? Or do you have neurotic tendencies?

How personality type and skincare are related is unclear; nonetheless, it seems that both women's skin and soul flaws will soon be out in the open!

Smart Mirror Virtual Try-On Make-Up

The virtual try-on experience might be the most exciting and cost-effective technological development in cosmetics. Smart mirror technology is astounding. The consumer can turn the head, flick the hair or even move around. The make-up and accessories stay in place because of what manufacturers call 'precise facial-point detection'.

Consumers describe the smart mirror as magical, super realistic, and a money-saving tool. Not surprisingly, it has become a shopping adventure for many women. Busy career women find they save time by cutting out travel and queues. Many younger women love experimenting with different products: foundation, blusher, lip colours, and eye products.

The smart mirror also enables the consumer to try out accessories: Younger consumers love trying on hair accessories and sunglasses. Career women prefer trying on trendy frames for reading glasses. Through smart mirror technology, the consumer has access to various products to choose from without leaving her home or wasting money on products that disappoint.

3D Bioprinting to Produce Human Tissue

3D printing is not new but has been used in many industries such as manufacturing, architecture, art, and design. The medical use of bioprinting involves several medical fields: stem cell biology, genetics, genomics, tissue engineering, nanotechnology, transplantation, and prosthetic bioengineering.

Printing human tissue is an exciting and complex new science to replace badly injured tendons, ligaments, or discs. It also holds immense possibilities for many other medical fields. For instance, it is expected that 3D bioprinting will soon eliminate drug testing on human volunteers and animals. It will replace human organ donors and prevent cell rejection within a few years.

But what is 3D bioprinting? In short, a person's stem cells are harvested from their fat cells. These are printed on hydrogel to create a structure on which living cells multiply, and even blood vessels are generated.

Stem cells, present in all human organs, are vital for recovery after an injury or operation. They are unique because they can be stimulated to develop into any tissue type, making them ideal for bioprinting different human tissue types. It means that stem cells taken from adipose tissue can, for instance, develop into cartilage to replace a nose or an ear.

To the layperson, laboratory-grown 3D body parts and organs sound like science fiction. Rightly so, as bioprinting and its applications in the medical field is an advanced and complicated science. It will still take some time to become generally available. It will eventually cause significant changes in the medical industry. Surgeons' education will dramatically change over the following decades. Bioprinting will have substantial financial implications as it requires high-tech, costly equipment.

Regenerative medicine is a challenging field with many safety concerns, such as contamination, toxicity, and cell safety. Still, bioprinting opens new possibilities for reconstructive and plastic surgery.

Bio inks use polysaccharides, protein, and synthetic polymers to recreate human skin to treat scars. Laboratory-grown living skin with three layers for burn wounds is already in the pipeline. Doctors will soon treat the white patches of vitiligo patients with growth factors, stem cells, and melanocytes.

In the cosmetic industry, facial recognition designs a facemask that fits tight on the face and prevents valuable products from running out.

Many advanced medical applications are still in development, and it will be a while before 3D bioprinting is readily available at your local plastic surgeon's office.

Penetration of the Stratum Corneum

Cosmetic products are a combination of active ingredients and their carriers. Active ingredients are discussed in Chapter 3. They have a specific action or work in the skin. Carriers are emulsions that form the vehicle by which the active ingredient is transported. To complicate matters further, skincare products come in various forms: liquid, gels, creams, or lotions.

Topical creams and lotions could potentially penetrate the skin through three pathways:

- The hair follicle could be a little reservoir for the active component for further distribution through the network of blood capillaries.

- Nanoparticles of active ingredients could possibly pass through the minute openings between the corneocytes (dead keratinocytes) and the lipid layer (consisting of fatty acids, ceramides, and cholesterol).

- A third possible pathway is transcellular penetration, where the active component is directly deposited in the living skin cells.

Nanotechnology

The nanometer scale is the smallest scale in the world; one nanometer is a billionth of a metre (Wikipedia). Nanotechnology is the science of things so small that the human eye can barely see them.

Nanotechnology has been around since 1986 (Salvioni, 2021). It has already improved skincare in numerous ways: deeper penetration through the skin barrier, more stable skincare ingredients, improved moisturising, and sunscreen lotions.

For decades, scientists have experimented with various techniques to get active ingredients through the brick-like stratum corneum. Nanoparticles might be the answer. Look at the pores on your skin, and the connection is clear: Nanotechnology in skincare can deliver delicate and small particles that might penetrate the skin barrier.

The ideal is that minute particles of bioactive components are deposited deep in the skin to enhance cellular renewal and collagen production. Direct deposits of active ingredients in the basal layer of the epidermis and the dermis can effectively address anti-ageing, dryness, and pigmentation.

The future of nanoparticles in products depends on scientists discovering nano substances that can penetrate, stabilise, and control the release of the active ingredient.

Penetration Enhancers

Although nanotechnology is making good progress, several studies on the skin barrier also try to penetrate this tough outer layer of the skin. Researchers in both the medical and cosmeceutical fields have worked tirelessly to find a solution for penetrating the skin barrier. Several drugs are applied topically, and better penetration and absorption will improve effectiveness. Cosmeceutical science similarly wants to deliver active ingredients deep into the skin.

Experts work on modifying the lipids in the skin barrier to allow for better absorption and penetration of active ingredients. The aim is to increase the moisture content of the lipid matrix between the dead corneocytes. The lipid construction in the stratum corneum can potentially be a pathway for active ingredients to be transported to the deeper skin layers. Research on carrier substances, usually oil or water-based, to transport active ingredients will further improve penetration enhancers.

Scientists report that they have to consider individual skin structures – thickness, lipid content, and enzyme activity – as these play a role in the ability of chemical enhancers to penetrate the stratum corneum. Because of various individual factors, one product cannot serve all skin types.

Also, enhancers are more effective in high concentrations, often irritating skin. The danger of irritations prompted experts to investigate the combination of devices discussed in Chapter 9 and chemical enhancers in low concentrations.

Physical Enhancers

Chapter 9 overviews physical enhancers, machines, and devices that work with electrical currents, lights, lasers, ultrasound, and many more. Over the last decades, these devices and machines have successfully overcome the impenetrable skin barrier. Some create minute wounds on the skin that help the transfer of active ingredients. Others use heat deeper in the skin to stimulate skin regeneration.

New research concentrates on penetrating the hard top layer: the lipid matrix in the stratum corneum, improved active ingredients, carrier emulsions, state-of-the-art machines, and devices. The ideal would be a single enhancer that does not irritate the skin, improves skin quality, and also functions as a cosmetic. Experts are hopeful that new technology will soon find a solution for penetrating the tough skin barrier without any danger of exposing the skin to outside viruses and bacteria.

High-Tech Surgery Techniques

Smart Lipo uses laser technology to heat and melt fat in a targeted area, such as the saddlebags on the hips. Experts assert it is much easier to remove liquified fat through suction.

An endoscopic facelift uses small incisions behind the hairline above the ear. The surgeon uses a flexible tube with a light and a camera to tighten the muscles in places where a traditional facelift could not reach: the frown line between the eyes, the folds along the nose, and the cheeks.

Current invasive surgical research concentrates on making surgery safer and more durable. It involves long-term involvement with patients to determine which techniques and methods can withstand the test of time. The skill to remove loose skin is constantly developed to lessen scarring and also to ensure the scar does not change position as the patient ages.

Surgeons use the term 'form and function' in removing excess skin. It is senseless to remove the skin from the upper arms to the extent that the patient can barely use the arm afterward. The same applies to removing excess skin from the upper eyelid. It can result in a patient not being able to close the eye properly when sleeping. Modern surgical research strives to determine the parameters of getting the best form without interfering with function (Toogood, 2022).

Quick Reminder

In the light of climate change and its imminent dangers, 21st-century consumers hold cosmeceutical companies responsible for sustainability in production, products, and packaging.

The skincare market is dynamic and responds to global economic and population needs. The bulk of sales has moved from the traditional western markets to Asia and Africa.

The demand for skincare has significantly increased. The cosmetic market is still growing but at a slower rate.

Africa has the biggest demand for cosmetics.

Because of the environmental impact of the petrochemical industry, biocosmetics are replacing fossil-based products.

Since the global pandemic, artificial intelligence has grown and will continue to do so. Online cosmetic sales are just the beginning. Women can and will progressively use artificial intelligence for skin analysis, identifying conditions and problems, determining treatments, and buying appropriate products.

Bioprinting is changing the face of many medical fields and opens new possibilities for regenerative and plastic surgery.

Penetration of the stratum corneum still limits the effectiveness of skincare products. Researchers aim to develop ingredients and methods to deliver active ingredients into the deeper layers of the skin.

Nanotechnology works toward nano substances that can penetrate, stabilise, and control the release of the active ingredients in the basal layer of the epidermis and also in the dermis.

Penetration enhancers complement nanotechnology and concentrate on the stratum corneum's lipid matrix to improve the absorption and transfer of the active ingredients to the lower skin layers.

Plastic surgery works endlessly to improve the safety and durability of surgery. It strives to lessen scarring, improve form and function, and balance the aesthetic with practical function.

Conclusion

The skin, in all its complexity, is the central theme of this guide. It is the most visible part of the human body, a non-verbal communicator, a beauty asset, and even a political weapon. It has the unique ability to renew itself constantly. Without words, the skin speaks and reveals who we are, what we think, and how we care for ourselves.

It is thus no wonder that skincare is as old as the human race. Since Cleopatra bathed in milk in a tub on the River Nile, women ingeniously used whatever was available to take care of their skin: mud, urine, chicken droppings, garden plants from their gardens, and animal fat.

Since mediaeval times, women wanted white skin and used whatever they could find to lighten their faces. They even used make-up with lead, which is poisonous and dangerous. The misconception that white skin is desirable caused immense pain and became a highly sensitive and politicised issue.

Fortunately, the 21st century finally ended the perception that only white skin is beautiful. Celebrities and ordinary women of all skin tones and hair textures now celebrate their unique features.

Beauty has a history of political involvement: At the beginning of the 20th century, suffragettes in New York adopted red lipstick as a symbol of emancipation. This trend continued during the two world wars when women wore red lipstick and make-up to boost their morale. It was endorsed by the military in the United States and England: Women who joined the U.S. army wore Montezuma Red, and civilian ladies Victory Red.

British women with red lips also proudly defied Nazism and Hitler, who strongly disliked make-up.

However, the skin is, in the first place, an organ without which human life is impossible. Thin as it is, it consists of various layers, sub-layers, and components. Each of these components has a specific function. The complexity of the skin's structure and function contributes to many myths and misconceptions about the skin.

The biggest misconception is probably that the skin can absorb skincare products. Unfortunately, it is not true: The outermost layer of the skin, the stratum corneum, consists of dead cells and forms a brick wall that no cosmeceutical product can yet penetrate successfully.

This does not mean that you should stop using skincare products. On the contrary, science has proved that skincare is vital to seal in the skin's natural lipids. This guide will give you the necessary information about skincare ingredients, their functions, and how they contribute to a strong skin barrier and healthy skin.

Current research concentrates on penetrating the stratum corneum to deposit active ingredients deep into the skin. Researchers are constantly trying to overcome this obstacle, and penetration enhancers and nanotechnology will soon deliver skin ingredients to the basal layer of the epidermis and the dermis.

The most amazing fact about human skin is that it renews itself constantly. Women who have neglected their skin should take notice: You might have damaged your skin because of lifestyle choices such as smoking, drinking, a lack of exercise, and a diet high in sugars and fats, but all is not lost. Depending on your age, the skin cells in the dermis move upward to the skin surface (the stratum corneum) every 30 to 45 days.

Because your skin is a living and dynamic organ with the ability to renew itself, the symptoms of premature ageing, sun damage, wrinkling, and age spots can be lessened, if not reversed. The same principle applies to people with problematic skin conditions. Your skin has the potential to improve with the proper lifestyle and, very importantly, the right treatment.

The skin works in cycles, and no treatment will give quick results. Healing and renewal take time and depend entirely on the individual's commitment to stay out of the sun, live and eat healthily, and follow the targeted treatment.

This guide does not include any trendy ideas or promote any cosmetic brand. It explains in lay language the science behind skincare. Only when you understand how your skin works can you treat it intelligently and not chase after trends.

If readers take one thing from this guide, let it be to avoid sun damage to the skin. Experts agree that extended exposure to the sun might be the most significant factor in skin ageing. Furthermore, the sun contributes to many skin problems and interferes in treatments for acne, pigmentation, and electrolysis. Skin cancer is not discussed here, as this is not a medical guide, but the danger of prolonged UV radiation cannot be overstated. Many experts go so far as to say that if a woman uses only one skin product, it should be sunscreen.

The beauty industry is vast, and marketing gimmicks are confusing and costly. Advertisements use scientific terminology that impresses but, at the same time, confuses the consumer. This guide takes the guessing out of terminology and marketing buzzwords.

The most significant source of confusion in skincare is its ingredients and their function. This guide lists the most common ingredients and gives the scientific background, explaining what the consumer can realistically expect of them.

Collagen is the principal protein in the dermis, and its importance cannot be emphasised enough. It is constantly renewed when young, but collagen production slows with ageing. There is still no scientific evidence that collagen (peptide) supplements and topical applications are effective. However, research on collagen replenishment is ongoing and promising.

Hyaluronic acid is a vital ingredient in skincare, and many advertisements emphasise its importance. It is a humectant that binds with water. Consequently, it effectively seals the skin surface and retains moisture. However, like other ingredients, hyaluronic acid cannot penetrate the stratum corneum.

Very few women have normal skin, and even fewer have flawless skin. Most women struggle with a skin problem at some stage of their lives. Knowing your skin and type is half the solution to skin issues. It should not be a guessing game.

This guide addresses the most common skin problems: pigmentation, acne, unwanted hair, tattoo regret, cellulite, sun damage, and ageing. Each of these is a complicated condition that can cause severe emotional distress and even social isolation. With knowledge about the causes, presentation, and treatment options, you will be able to self-treat or know when professional help is necessary.

Dermatologists use scientific methods to treat skin problems, and no woman needs to hide away because of a skin condition.

Based on the skin's reaction to sunburn, the Fitzpatrick skin qualification system has been used for many decades to determine the individual's chances of getting skin cancer.

Baumann's system helps to determine the skin's properties based on the skin's tendency to be oily versus dry, sensitive versus resistant, pigmented versus non-pigmented, and wrinkle-prone versus wrinkle-resistant.

The Roberts scale determines the individual's type of hyperpigmentation and the probability of long-term scarring because of pigmentation.

The 21st century and climate change brought a new dimension to skincare. Globally, consumers are concerned about the environment and expect the beauty industry to deliver on sustainability without compromising product quality.

Biocosmetics will eventually replace fossil-based ingredients, but consumers demand transparency in production and packaging.

The COVID-19 pandemic opened the door to online shopping, and manufacturers did more than just deliver products at the front door. Artificial intelligence made skin analysis, treatment options, and virtual make-up trials possible. The future of skincare undeniably includes the continued development of intelligent software and tools to provide personalised skincare.

Bioprinting brought exciting developments in the medical and beauty industry. It promises laboratory-grown ligaments, tendons, and even organs. Surgeons already create 3D prints of the human skin to treat scars and burn wounds. It opens many possibilities for bioprinting applications in cosmetic and regenerative surgery.

This guide challenges you to embrace your unique beauty and ethnic skin. It will help you to identify your skin problem and find a solution.

Celebrate who you are, know your skin, and understand the science behind skin ingredients. Beauty is diverse; beauty is not trying to adhere to trends or be eternally young. Live your reality, but be the best version of yourself at every stage of your life.

You are worth it.

References

AAFE American Academy of Facial Esthetics. (n.d.). *Dentists doing botox? It's about time.* https://www.facialesthetics.org/dentists-botox-time/

Abelmann, D. (2020 February 20). *What is toner, anyway?* Allure.https://www.allure.com/story/what-is-toner

Acme-Hardesty. (n.d.). *Green cosmetics: The push for sustainable beauty.* https://www.acme-hardesty.com/green-cosmetics-sustainable-beauty/

Alberts, B., Johnson, A., Lewis, J. et al. (2002). Fibroblasts and their transformations: the connective-tissue cell family. Molecular *Biology of the Cell,* Edition 4. National Library of Medicine. https://www.ncbi.nlm.nih.gov

Alex, A. (2016 October 9). *Cleopatra, queen of ancient Egypt, took baths in donkey milk to preserve her beauty and youth.* The Vintage News. https://www.thevintagenews.com/2016/10/09/said-cleopatra-queen-ancient-egypt-took-baths-donkey-milk-preserve-beauty-youth-skin-2

Alitura (2021 April 20). *The worst for your skin: How polyunsaturated fats age skin.* Alitura International. https://alitura.com/blogs/beauty-benefits/the-worst-oils-for-your-skin-how-polyunsaturated-fats-age-skin

Almarill. (2020). *Learn about the different types of skin.* https://www.almarill.com/your-health/your-skin/types-of-skin/

Ambardekar, N. (2021 November 3). *Slideshow: Surprising ways smoking affects your looks and life.* WebMD. https://www.webmd.com/smoking-cessation/ss/slideshow-ways-smoking-affects-looks

Anderson, L. (2021 September 20). *The 10 most common skin conditions.* Drugs.com. https://www.drugs.com/slideshow/most-common-skin-conditions-1086

Arné. (n.d.). *LED it shine: How NASA throws some light on your skin.* https://arneskincare.com/blogs/news/led-it-shine

Arora, G. & Arora, S. (2019 July - September). Neck rejuvenation with thread lift. *Journal of Cutaneous and Aesthetic Surgery.* https://www.ncbi.nlm.nih.gov/pmc/articles/PMC6785971/

Astanza. (2022). *How laser tattoo removal works.* https://astanzalaser.com/wp-content/uploads/2017/08/eBook3.pdf

Axtell, B. (2020 September 2). *Cellulite.* WebMD. https://www.webmd.com/beauty/get-rid-of-cellulite

Ayurvedic Professionals UK. (2020). *Ayurveda in UK.* https://www.aapuk.net/ayurveda-in-uk

Baird, M. L. (2021 March 11). 'Making Black more beautiful.' Black women and the cosmetics industry in the Post-civil Rights Era. *Gender & History.* https://onlinelibrary.wiley.com/doi/full/10.1111/1468-0424.12522

Balsamo, L. (2021 May 24). *Clean beauty has a misinformation problem.* Cosmopolitan. https://www.cosmopolitan.com/style-beauty/beauty/a36332134/clean-and-natural-beauty-myths/

Barber DTS. (2022). *Tattoo Needle Guide.* https://www.barberdts.com/uk/advice-hub/tattoo-needle-guide/

Baumann, L. (2014 September). *A novel approach to understanding the skin type.* ResearchGate. https://www.researchgate.net/publication/288321555

Baumann, L. (2008). Understanding and treating various skin types: The Baumann Skin Indicator. *Dermatologic Clinics,* Volume 26. Issue 3. https://pubmed.ncbi.nlm.nih.gov/18555952/

Baumann, L. (n.d.). https://lesliebaumannmd.com/#skintypesolutions

Baumann, L., Bernstein, E. F., Daniels, R. (2021 September 3). Clinical relevance of elastin in the structure and function of the skin. *Aesthetic Surgery Journal.* https://academic.oup.com/asjopenforum/article/3/3/ojab019/6275566

Baxter, H. (n.d.). *Which laser treatment is the best for your hyperpigmentation?* Coveteur. https://coveteur.com/2020/04/14/hyperpigmentation-laser-treatment/

Beijing Tourism. (2016 November 8). *Skincare in Ancient China.* ttps://english.visitbeijing.com.cn/article/47ONhI0YZ1T

Bellissimo. (n.d.). *Electrolysis Treatment: Preparation and after-care.* Bellissimo Skin & Body. https://www.bellissimoskin.co.nz/news/electrolysis-treatment-preparation-and-after-care/

Berman, R. (2022 June 9). *'Gender-affirming hormone therapy is life-saving,' expert says.* MedicalNewsToday. https://www.medicalnewstoday.com/articles/gender-affirming-hormone-therapy-is-life-saving-expert-says

Best Health. (2022 January 19). *The truth about petroleum: Does it belong in your skincare products?* Best Health Magazine. https://www.besthealthmag.ca/article/the-truth-about-petrolatum/

Bhattacharya, S. (2022 January 21). *8 Side effects of everyday makeup and what you can do about it.* Skinkraft. https://skinkraft.com/blogs/articles/side-effects-of-wearing-makeup-everyday

Biswas, S., Das, R., Banerjee, E. R. (2017 October 25). Role of free radicals in human inflammatory diseases. *Biophysics.* https://pdfs.semanticscholar.org/4a54/7cf946de313e7 0e8e1e53186d22e337288bd.pdf

Borkow, G. (2014 August 8). Using copper to improve the well-being of the skin. *Current Chemical Biology.* PubMed Central. https://www.ncbi.nlm.nih.gov/pmc/articles/PMC4556 990/

Bowman, J. (2020 July 30). *The 4 best vitamins for your skin.* Healthline. https://www.healthline.com/health/4-best-vitamins-for-skin#talk-to-your-doctor

Brainy Quotes. (n.d.). https://www.brainyquote.com/topics/rituals-quotes

Brown, D. (2020 December 7). *Latest innovations and technology in the field of plastic surgery.* SWAAY. https://swaay.com/latest-innovations-and-technology-in-the-field-of-plastic-surgery

Brown University. (2004 June 4). Insulin plays central role in aging, Brown scientists discover. *ScienceDaily.* www.sciencedaily.com/releases/2004/06/04060306493 5.htm

Burgess, L. (2020 June 23). *Which Fitzpatrick skin type are you?* MedicalNewsToday. https://www.medicalnewstoday.com/articles/320639# fitzpatrick-skin-types

Cancer Research UK. (2021 March 9). *Does hormone replacement therapy (HRT) increase cancer risk?* https://www.cancerresearchuk.org/about-cancer/causes-of-cancer/hormones-and-cancer/does-hormone-replacement-therapy-increase-cancer-risk

Cao, C., Xiao, Z., Wu, Y. et al. (2020 March 12). Diet and skin aging – from the perspective of food nutrition. *Nutrients MDPI.* https://www.ncbi.nlm.gov/pmc/articles/PMC7146365

Cartwright, M. (2013 October 10). Montezuma. *World History Encyclopedia. https://www.worldhistory.org/Montezuma/*

CDC. (2022 June 27). *Cellulitis: All you need to know.* Centers for Disease Control and Prevention. https://www.cdc.gov/groupastrep/diseases-public/Cellulitis.html

Charter, C. (2019 January 21). *Are cosmetics bad for the environment?* Botanical Trader. https://botanicaltrader.com/blogs/news/how-your-beauty-products-are-killing-coral-reefs-turtles-rainforests-more

Cherney, K. (2019 March 19). *About skin pH and why it matters.* Healthline. https://www.healthline.com/health/whats-so-important-about-skin-ph

Cherney, K. (2019 March 7). *Everything you need to know about using alpha-hydroxy acids (AHAs)*. Healthline. https://www.healthline.com/health/beauty-skin-care/alpha-hydroxy-acid

Cherney, K. (2022 March 7). 8 *Options for Hyperpigmentation*. Healthline. https://www.healthline.com/health/beauty-skin-care/hyperpigmentation-treatment

Chertoff, J. (n.d.). *Stem cells in skin care: What they do and how they work*. Dermstore. https://www.dermstore.com/blog/stem-cells-in-skin-care/

Chung, J. (2022 April 7). *The (un)regulation of tattoo ink*. The Regulatory Review. https://www.theregreview.org/2022/04/07/chung-unregulation-of-tattoo-ink/

Cleveland Clinic (2020 April 12). *Actinic keratosis*. https://my.clevelandclinic.org/health/diseases/14148-actinic-keratosis

Cleveland Clinic. (2022 May 5). *Ance papules: What are Acne papules?* https://my.clevelandclinic.org/health/diseases/22905-acne-papules

Cleveland Clinic: (2021 December 11). *Blackheads: What are blackheads?* https://my.clevelandclinic.org/health/diseases/22038-blackheads

Cleveland Clinic. (2021 October 28). *Cellulite*. https://my.clevelandclinic.org/health/diseases/17694-cellulite

Cleveland Clinic. (2021 August 25). *Cystic acne: What is cystic acne?* https://my.clevelandclinic.org/health/diseases/21737-cystic-acne

Cleveland Clinic. (2021 May 1). *Electrolysis.* https://my.clevelandclinic.org/health/treatments.8306-electrolysis

Cleveland Clinic. (2021 August 24). *Facelift (Rhytidectomy).* https://my.clevelandclinic.org/health/treatments/11023-facelift

Cleveland Clinic. (2021 November 13). *Facial Muscles.* https://my.clevelandclinic.org/health/body/21672-facial-muscles

Cleveland Clinic. (2022 April 4). *Hormonal imbalances.* https://my.clevelandclinic.org/health/diseases/22673-hormonal-imbalance

Cleveland Clinic. (2021 July 21). *Inflammation.* https://my.clevelandclinic.org/health/symptoms/21660-inflammation

Cleveland Clinic. (2022 May 2). *Nodular Acne: What they look like.* https://my.clevelandclinic.org/health/diseases/22888-nodular-acne

Cleveland Clinic. (n.d.) *Skin diseases.* https://my.clevelandclinic.org/health/diseases/21573-skin-diseases

Cleveland Clinic. (2021 November 2). *The truth about dry brushing and what it does for you.* https://health.clevelandclinic.org/the-truth-about-dry-brushing-and-what-it-does-for-you/

Cleveland Clinic. (2022 February 24). *Vitamin E for skin: What does it do?* https://health.clevelandclinic.org/vitamin-e-for-skin-health

Clinical Applications of Scientific Innovation. (2019 August 22). *The underappreciated role of elevated insulin in skin disorders.* https://blog.designsforhealth.com/node/1089

Colihan, K. (2008 July 21). *Removing tattoos: Who does it and why?* WebMD. https://www.webmd.com/skin-problems-and-treatments/news/20080721/removing-tattoos-who-does-it-and-why

Come Step Back In Time. (2014 August 4). *Perfumes, compacts & powders – Francois Coty & the Doughboys: Stories from the Great War Part 10.* https://comestepbackintime.wordpress.com/2014/08/09/perfumes-compacts-powders-francois-coty-the-doughboys-stories-from-the-great-war-part-10/

Craig, M. L. (2017 November 20). Black women and beauty culture in the 20th-century America. *Oxford Research Encyclopedia.* https://oxfordre.com/americanhistory/americanhistory/view/10.1093/acrefore/9780199329175.001.0001/acrefore-9780199329175-e-433

Davidson, K. (2022 April 15). *Is it possible to get rid of cellulite with exercises?* Healthline. https://www.healthline.com/health/fitness-exercise/cellulite-exercises#workout-plan

Deana. (n.d.). *Innovative trends and technology in beauty and skincare industry.* Innovative Cloud. https://innovationcloud.com/blog/innovative-trends-and-technology-in-beauty-and-skincare-industry.html

De Soto, L. (2022 March 31). *Does selenium really slow aging?* MedicalNewsToday. https://www.medicalnewstoday.com/articles/does-selenium-really-slow-aging

DFW Anti-Aging (2020 January 24). *Which hormones make you look younger?* DFW Anti-Aging Wellness Centers https://www.dfwantiagingwellness.com/2020/01/24/which-hormones-make-you-look-younger

Dix, M. (2019 September 29). *Everything you should know about oxidative stress.* Healthline. https://www.healthline.com/health/oxidative-stress

Drakati, E., Dessinioti, C., Antoniou, C. V. (2014 May 15). Air pollution and the skin. *Frontiers in Environmental Science,* https://www.frontiersin.org/articles/10.3389/

Dreno, B., Bagatin, E., Blume-Peytavi, U. et al. (2018 September 14). Female type of adult acne: Physiological and psychological consideration and management. *Journal of German Society of Dermalotology.*https://onlinelibrary.wiley.com/doi/full/10.1111/ddg.13664

Duffill, M. (2008). *Dermatosis papulosa nigra.* Dermnet NZ. https://dermnetnz.org/topics/dermatosis-papulosa-nigra

Dunmade, O. (2022 May 4). 5 *Ancient beauty rituals.* Pulse.ng. https://www.pulse.ng/lifestyle/beauty-health/5-ancient-african-beauty-rituals/3d64vr4

Ecowatch. (2016 May 6). *5 Ways Eating Processed Foods Messes with Your Body* https://www.ecowatch.com/5-ways-eating-processed-foods-messes-with-your-body-1891128657.html

Eilers, S., Bach, D. Q., Gaber, R. et al. (2013 November). Accuracy of self-report in assessing Fitzpatrick Skin Phototypes 1 through to VI. *JAMA Dermatology*. https://jamanetwork.com/journals/jamadermatology/fullarticle/1727180

Electrolysis Beauty Lounge. (n.d.). *The history of electrolysis*. https://www.electrolysisbeautylounge.com/history-of-electrolysis

Ellis, M. E. (2017 December 24). *Liver spots (solar lentiginosis)*. Healthline. https://www.healthline.com/health/liver-spots

Ellis, R. R. (2022 February 17). *CoolSculpting*. WebMD. https://www.webmd.com/beauty/coolsculpting

E Medical Clinic. (2021 November 1). *Do topical peptides (AKA skincare) work?* https://e-medicalclinic.com/topical-peptides-aka-skincare-work/

EPA. (2022 March 7). *Endocrine Disruption What is the endocrine system?* United States Environmental Protection Agency. ps://www.epa.gov/endocrine-disruption/what-endocrine-system

Eske, J. (2020 December 14). *What is Sebum?* MedicalNewsToday. https://www.medicalnewstoday.com/articles/sebum#summary

Eucerin. (2022). *How does skin differ by ethnic group?* https://www.en.eucerin-me.com/about-skin-knowledge/skin-ethnics

Eucerin. (2022). *Hyperpigmentation – What causes dark spots and how can I reduce them?* https://int.eucerin.com/skin-concerns/uneven-skin/hyperpigmentation

Eucerin. (2022). *Post-inflammatory hyperpigmentation – What causes it and how can I reduce it?* https://int.eucerin.com/about-skin/indications/hyperpigmentation-caused-by-inflammation

F. C. Simple Skincare Science. (2019 March 7). *Why science says hyaluronic acid is the holy grail to wrinkle-free, youthful hydration.* Simple Skincare Science. https://www.healthline.com/health/beauty-skin-care/hyaluronic-acid

FDA. (2022). *Tattoos & permanent makeup: Fact Sheet.* https://www.fda.gov/cosmetics/cosmetic-products/tattoos-permanent-makeup-fact-sheet

Fjermedal, G. (2022 May 24). *Smart makeup mirror & AR try-on real-world applications.* https://www.perfectcorp.com/business/blog/commerce/how-beauty-tech-is-revolutionizing-the-customer-experience

Fletcher, J. (2018 August 2). *What happens when a woman has low testosterone?* MedicalNewsToday. https://www.medicalnewstoday.com/articles/322663

Fleur & Bee. (2021 April 16). *Preservatives in skincare: Are they safe?* https://fleurandbee.com/blogs/news/preservatives-in-skin-care

Florida Dermatology. (2020 January 23). *How stress affects your skin.* Floria Dermatology and Skin Cancer Centers. https://fldscc.com/2020/01/23/how-stress-affects-skin/

Florida Dermatology. (2021 October 31). *What does sugar do to your skin?* Florida Dermatology and Skin Cancer

Centers. https://fldscc.com/2021/10/31/what-does-sugar-do-to-skin/

Frey, F. (2021 October 27). *Skin Care products: False claims and broken promises at your expense.* 50plustoday. https://50plus-today.com/false-claims-skin-care/

Fried, R. G. (2013 September). Acne vulgaris: The psychological & physiological burden of illness. *Dermatologist.* https://www.hmpgloballearningnetwork.com/site/the derm/site/cathlab/event/acne-vulgaristhe-psychosocial-and-psychological-burden-illness

Fulghum Bruce, D. (2022 May 4). *Normal testosterone and estrogen levels in women.* WebMD. https://www.webmd.com/women/guide/normal-testosterone-and-estrogen-levels-in-women

Ganceviciene, R., Liakou, A., Yheodoridis, A. et al. (20112 July 1). Skin anti-aging strategies. *Dermato Endocrinology* 4(3). https://www.ncbi.nlm.nih.gov/pmc/articles/PMC3583 892/

Gardner, C. (2022 July 20). *Linda Evangelista settles CoolSculpting suit after "horrific ordeal" with cosmetic procedure.* The Hollywood Reporter. https://www.hollywoodreporter.com/lifestyle/lifestyle-news/linda-evangelista-coolsculpting-suit-settled-disfigured-1235183868/

Gardner, S. (2022 January 17). 5 *Signs and symptoms of psoriasis.* WebMD. https://www.webmd.com/skin-problems-and-treatments/psoriasis/psoriasis-signs-symptoms

Gardner, S. (2020 March 29). *Conditions that can cause body hair loss.* WebMD. https://www.webmd.com/a-to-z-guides/ss/slideshow-body-hair-loss-causes

Gardner, S. (2022 April 22). *Laser tattoo removal: What to know.* WebMD. https://www.webmd.com/skin-problems-and-treatments/laser-tattoo-removal

Gardner, S. (2022 April 26). *Skin conditions and warts.* WebMD. https://www.webmd.com/skin-problems-and-treatments/warts

Geng, K. (2022 March 17). *What is organic skincare and how is it different?* MedicalNewsToday. https://www.medicalnewstoday.com/articles/organic-skin-care

Ghansiyal, A. (2021 January 12). *Mud baths and everything you wanted to know about them.* Travel.earth. https://travel.earth/everything-you-wanted-to-know-about-mud-baths/

Giacomoni, P. U. (2005 July 6). Ageing, science and the cosmetics industry. *EMBO Reports Supplement* 1. tps://www.ncbi.nlm.nih.gov/pmc/articles/PMC1369266/

Ginn, L. (2009 October 10). *Ethnic skin types.* Skinsights. https://www.skinsight.com/health-topics/ethnic-skin-types

González-Minero, F. J., Bravo-Días, L. (2018 August 19). The use of plants in skin-care products, cosmetics and fragrances: Past and present. *Cosmetics.* https://www.mdpi.com/2079-9284/5/3/50

Gorman, M. O., Miller, K. (2020 June 11). *8 Things your body hair says about your health, according to doctors.* Prevention. https://www.prevention.com/health/a20467472/body-hair-causes/

Gosling, L. (2013 December 16). Saving face - *Beauty for Women Workers during the First World War.* https://blog.maryevans.com/2013/12/saving-face-beauty-for-women-workers-during-the-first-world-war.html

Go-TelAviv.com. (2012). *The incredible Dead Sea.* https://www.go-telaviv.com/dead-sea-history.html

Gov.UK. (2020 December 31). *Guidance: Organic food: UK-approved control bodies.* https://www.gov.uk/guidance/organic-food-uk-approved-control-bodies

Goyal, N., Jerold, F. (2021 November 25). Biocosmetics: technological advances and future outlook. *Springer Link.* https://link.springer.com/article/10.1007/s11356-021-17567-3

Grant, E.T. (2018 October 3). *The 7 most common tattoos women get removed, according to laser surgeons.* Bustle.https://www.bustle.com/p/the-7-most-common-tattoos-women-get-removed-according-to-laser-surgeons-12121101

Guha, A. (n.d.). *Where does Ayurveda come from?* Earl E. Bakken Center for Spirituality and Healing. https://www.takingcharge.csh.umn.edu/where-ayurveda-come-from

Gunnars, K. (2019 May 23). *What are Omega-3 fatty acids? Explained in simple terms.* Healthline. https://www.healthline.com/nutrition/what-are-omega-3-fatty-acids

HadeethEnc.com. (n.d.). *Hadith.* https://hadeethenc.com/en/browse/hadith/10036

Halcyon Dermatology. (n.d.). *Platelet-rich plasma (PRP) facial rejuvenation.* https://www.halcyonderm.com/cosmetic/skin-body-treatments/prp-facial-rejuvenation/

Hamilton, T., De Gannes, G. (2011 April 16). *Allergic contact dermatitis to preservatives and fragrances in cosmetics.* PubMed. https://pubmed.ncbi.nlm.nih.gov/21611680/

Hammond, C. (2012 May 29). *Why having more pigment can help deal with, but not fully stop, the tell-tale signs of ageing skin.* BBC Future. https://www.bbc.com/future/article/20120529-does-darker-skin-not-wrinkle

Harvard Health Publishing, (2021 November 16). *Foods that fight inflammation.* https://www.health.harvard.edu/staying-healthy/foods-that-fight-inflammation

Hazell, K. (2011 December 29). *Blood vessels linked to menopausal hot flushes.* The Huffington Post UK. https://www.huffingtonpost.co.uk/2011/12/29/blood-vessels-linked-to-menopausal-hot-flushes

HealthEngine. (2010 November 4). *Cosmetic surgery: An introduction.* https://healthinfo.healthengine.com.au/cosmetic-surgery-an-introduction

Heath, E. (2021 July 12). *Natural vs. synthetic cosmetics ingredients: What are they and what's the difference?* Goldn. https://goldn.com/blog/posts/natural-vs-synthetic-cosmetics-ingredients-what-are-they/

Hecht, M. (2019 March 4). *What are the Fitzpatrick skin types?* Healthline.

https://www.healthline.com/health/beauty-skin-care/fitzpatrick-skin-types

History.com Editors. (2022 March 15). *Madam C. J. Walker.* History.com. https://www.history.com/topics/black-history/madame-c-j-walker

History Undressed. (2008 March 10). *Historical methods of hair removal.* https://www.historyundressed.com/2008/03/ladies-have-you-ever-forgotten-to-shave.html

Honigmann, M. (2021 December 16). *What are parabens? The truth about skincare's biggest bad guy.* Elle. https://www.elle.com/uk/beauty/skin/articles/a36356/what-are-parabens/

Howley. L. (2022 June 28). *5 Reasons why brands need futuristic skincare technology.* https://www.perfectcorp.com/business/blog/ai-skincare/5-reasons-why-skincare-brands-need-to-adopt-ai-technology

Hullett, A. (2022 May 23). *Can cupping really smooth out cellulite?* https://greatist.com/health/cupping-for-cellulite

Hunter, D. (2019 August 12). *Why do people get tattoos?* Authority Tattoo. https://authoritytattoo.com/why-do-people-get-tattoos/

Ink & Water Tattoo. (n.d.). *How do machines work?* https://www.inkandwatertattoo.ca/how-tattoo-machines-work

Inmode (2020 March 18). *The latest innovations in cellulite treatments.* https://www.inmode.com.au/blogs/news/the-latest-innovations-in-cellulite-treatments

Innovations Medical. (n.d.). *Diet to get rid of cellulite.* https://innovationsmedical.com/diet-to-get-rid-of-cellulite/

Institute BCN (2022). Ginkgo Biloba. https://institutebcn.com/en/classics/ginkgo-biloba/

Isaacs, T. (2012 March). Skin hypersensitivity reactions to preservatives. *Current Allergy and Clinical Immunology.* The University of Cape Town. https://journals.co.za/doi/pdf/10.10520/EJC120042

Jacob, B. (2022 April 18). *The revival of ancient beauty rituals.* BBC Culture. https://www.bbc.com/culture/article/20220408-the-revival-of-ancient-beauty-rituals

Jaliman, D. (2021 August 7). *Hyperpigmentation, hypopigmentation, and your skin.* WebMD. https://www.webmd.com/skin-problems-and-treatments/hyperpigmentation-hypopigmentation

Jaret, P. (2011 April 15) *Exercise for healthy skin.* WebMD. https://www.webmd.com/skin-problems-and-treatments/acne/features/exercise

Jennings, K-A. (2021 July 3). 5 *Science-based benefits of niacin (Vitamin B3)* Healthline. https://www.healthline.com/nutrition/niacin-benefits

Jesitus, J. (2019 June 12). *Inflammation and aging.* Dermatology Times. https://www.dermatologytimes.com/view/inflammation-and-aging

John Hopkins Medicine. (n.d.). *Acne.* https://www.hopkinsmedicine.org/health/conditions-and-diseases/acne

John Hopkins Medicine. (n.d.). *Ayurveda.* https://www.hopkinsmedicine.org/health/wellness-and-prevention/ayurveda

Joi, S. (2009 March 4). *The rare body tricks only some of us can do.* Glamour. https://www.glamour.com/story/wiggle-your-ears-raise-one-eye

Jones, D. (2019 February 19) *Electrolysis the business.* Positive Pathways Beauty and Cosmetic Services.

Jones, N. (2014 June 19). *'Breaking up is hard 'Tattoo': 7 celebs who have removed their ex-themed ink.* People. https://people.com/celebrity/angelina-jolie-melanie-griffith-and-more-stars-who-have-removed-tattoos/

Jovic, T., Jessop, Z. & Whitaker, I. (2018 January) 3D Bioprinting for surgical reconstruction and organ transplantation. *ResearchGate.* https://www.researchgate.net/publication/327344757_3D_Bioprinting_for_Surgical_Reconstruction_and_Organ_Transplantation

Julson, E. (2018 January 24). *Top 7 foods that can cause acne.* Healthline. https://www.healthline.com/nutrition/foods-that-cause-acne

Khan Academy. (n.d.). *Responses to the environment: Animal Communication.* https://www.khanacademy.org/science/ap-biology/ecology-ap/responses-to-the-environment/a/animal-communication

Kahn, A. (2019 July 31). *What causes pustules?* Healthline. https://www.healthline.com/health/pustules

Kam, K. (2011 April 15). *Medications that can cause acne.* WebMD. https://www.ncbi.nlm.nih.gov/pmc/articles/PMC7527 424/

Karim,R. (2012 November 9). Tattoo *Psychology: Art of self-destruction? Modern-day Social Branding.* HuffPost Contributor. https://www.huffpost.com/entry/psychology-of-tattoos_b_2017530

Kaus, J. (2021 July 19). *Seeing spots? Treating hyperpigmentation.* Mayo Clinic. https://www.aad.org/public/diseases/a-z/melasma-treatment

Kerns H. (2021 February 15). *The one food dermatologists never eat because it causes wrinkles & fine lines.* SheFinds. https://www.shefinds.com/collections/trans-fats-aging-skin/

Kester, S. (2021 March 19). *Skin elasticity: dermatologists share how to keep skin firm.* Vital Proteins. https://www.vitalproteins.com/blogs/beauty/skin-elasticity

Kim, B., Cho, H-E., Moon, S. H. et al. (2020 April 7). Transdermal delivery systems in cosmetic surgery. *Biomedical Dermatology* Volume 4 Article 10(2020). https://biomeddermatol.biomedcentral.com/articles/1 0.1186/s41702-020-0058-7

Kingsway. (2022). *Alcohol and aging effects: Does alcohol make you look older and cause wrinkles?* https://kingswayrecovery.com/alcohol-and-aging-effects/

Kitomba. (2022 February 1). *Industry insights: The effects of Covvid-19 on the hair and beauty industry in Q4 2021.* Kitomba Blog. https://www.kitomba.com/blog/industry-insights-the-effects-of-covid-19-on-the-hair-and-beauty-industry-in-q4-2021/

Kivi, R., Solan, M. (2021 September 22). *Understanding albinism.* Healthline. https://www.healthline.com/health/albinism

Kleszckynski, K.. Fischer T.W. (2012 July 1). Melatonin and human skin ageing. *Dermo Endrocornology.* https://www.ncbi.nlm.nih.gov/pmc/articles/PMC3583 885/

Kolarsick, P. A. J., Kolarskick, M. A. & Goodwin, C. (2011 July). Anatomy and Physiology of the skin. *Journal of Dermatology Nurses' Association,* Volume 3, Issue 4.

Kramer O. (2019 August 6). *Everything you need to know about whiteheads.* HealthLine. https://www.healthline.com/health/whitehead

Krant, J., (2017). *The role of collagen in skincare.* Art of Dermatology. https://artofdermatology.com/role-collagen-skin-care/

Kristic, M. (2021 January 17) *History of perfume: 24 Interesting facts and insights.* Scent Grail. https://scentgrail.com/scent-grail-learning-center/history-of-perfume/

Kunde, R. (2021 November 24). *What to know about ceramides for skin.* WebMD. https://www.webmd.com/beauty/what-to-know-about-ceramides-for-skin

Kwan, K. (2012 May 23). *4 Ways to put yourself first.* Sheknows https://www.sheknows.com/health-and-wellness/articles/1061439/how-to-put-yoursself-first-2/

Laneri. R. (2017 April 2). *The vicious rivalry between makeup's most powerful women ruined them.* New York Post. https://nypost.com/2017/04/02/the-vicious-rivalry-between-makeups-most-powerful-women-ruined-them/

Laseraway.com. (2019 January 14). *A brief history of skincare through the ages.* INB Medical. https://www.inbmedical.com/the-evolving-role-of-skincare

Lawton, S. (2019 November 11). Skin: The structure and functions of the skin. *Nursing Times.* https://www.webmd.com/skin-problems-and-treatments/hair-loss/science-hair

Leonard, J. (2019 October 16). *What to know about peptides for health.* MedicalNewsToday. https://www.medicalnewstoday.com/articles/326701

Lewis, K. (n.d.). Katie Lewis The Clinic. https://katielewis.uk/

Limoges Beauty. (n.d.). *How to get the best results from Electrolysis: Part 1.* http://topelectrolysisnyc.com/how-to-get-the-best-results-from-electrolysis-part-1/

Limoges Beauty. (n.d.). *How to get the best results from Electrolysis: Part 2.* http://topelectrolysisnyc.com/how-to-get-the-best-results-from-electrolysis-part-2/

Lister, T. (2012). *Optical properties of human skin.* SPIE Digital Library. http://www.spiedigitallibrary.org

Liu, C., Nassim, J. (2019 September 23). *Adult acne: Understanding underlying causes and banishing breakouts.* Harvard Health Publishing. https://www.health.harvard.edu/blog/adult-acne-

understanding-underlying-causes-and-banishing-
breakouts-2019092117816

Ludmann, P. (2022 February 15). *Melasma: Diagnosis and
treatment A to Z diseases.* American Academy of
Dermatology Association.
https://www.aad.org/public/diseases/a-z/melasma-
treatment

MacGill, M. (2018 July 23). *Hormonal acne: What you need to know.*
MedicalNewsToday.
https://www.medicalnewstoday.com/articles/313084

Macintyre K., Dobson, B. (2018 October). *Ochre: An ancient
health-giving cosmetic.* Anthropology from the shed.
https://anthropologyfromtheshed.com/project/ochre-
an-ancient-health-giving-cosmetic/

MacKay. B. (1989 May 26). *Hair Removal in history.* The
Washington Post.
https://www.washingtonpost.com/archive/lifestyle/19
89/05/26/hair-removal-in-history/

Malik, R. (2018 March 5). *Skin lightening – the lowdown.*
https://www.drrabiamalik.com/blogs/news/skin-
lightening-the-lowdown

Marks, D. H., Hagigeorges, D., Manatis-Lornell, A. J. et al.
(2019 September 25). Excess hair, hair removal
methods, and barriers to care in gender minority
patients: A survey study. *Journal of Cosmetic Dermatology.*
https://onlinelibrary.wiley.com/doi/epdf/10.1111/joc
d.13164

Martinez, P. (2022 May 3). *Environmental sustainability in the beauty
industry.* Unsustainable Magazine.
https://www.unsustainablemagazine.com/sustainability
-in-beauty-industry/

Mayo Clinic. (2022 January 21). *Chemical Peel.* https://www.mayoclinic.org/tests-procedures/chemical-peel/about/pac-20393473

Mayo Clinic. (2020 June 17). *Cold sore.* https://www.mayoclinic.org/diseases-conditions/cold-sore/symptoms-causes/syc-20371017

Mayo Clinic. (2022 May 4). *Cosmetic surgery.* https://www.mayoclinic.org/tests-procedures/cosmetic-surgery/about/pac-20385138

Mayo Clinic. (2022 June 3) *Hormone therapy: Is it right for you?* https://www.mayoclinic.org/diseases-conditions/menopause/in-depth/hormone-therapy/art-20046372

Mayo Clinic. (2022 May 4). *Laser hair removal.* https://www.mayoclinic.org/tests-procedures/laser-hair-removal/about/pac-20394555

Mayo Clinic. (2022 March 2). *laser resurfacing.* https://www.mayoclinic.org/tests-procedures/laser-resurfacing/about/pac-20385114

Mayo Clinic (2020 October 3). *Polycystic ovary syndrome. (PCOS).* https://www.mayoclinic.org/diseases-conditions/pcos/symptoms-causes/syc-20353439

McCormick, R. (2015 June 10). *Wonder at the science behind amazing skin.* Raconteur. https://www.raconteur.net/wonder-at-the-science-behind-amazing-skin/

McIntosh, J. (2017 June 16). *What is collagen, and why do people use it?* MedicalNewsToday. https://www.medicalnewstoday.com/articles/262881

McNeill, F. E. (2022 February 27). *Dying for makeup: Lead cosmetics posioned 18th-century European socialites in search of whiter skin.* The Conversation. https://theconversation.com/dying-for-makeup-lead-cosmetics-poisoned-18th-century-european-socialites-in-search-of-whiter-skin-176237

MeDermis Laser Clinic. (2022). *Tattoo ink safety: what are they made from?* https://medermislaserclinic.com/blog/what-are-tattoo-inks-made-from/

MedlinePlus. (n.d.). *Allergens.* National Library of Medicine. https://medlineplus.gov/article

Mehra, S. (2021 August 12). *Active ingredients 101: The what why and how.* Sublime Life. https://sublimelife.in/blogs/sublime-stories/active-ingredients-101-the-what-why-and-how

Melior. (2019 May 13). *Facial fat pads and their link to ageing.* https://www.meliorclinics.co.uk/blog/2019/05/13/facial-fat-pads-and-their-link-to-ageing/

Michalak, J. (2022 February 17). *Why has the popularity of tattoos grown?* Byrdie. https://www.byrdie.com/why-are-tattoos-popular-3189518

Migala, J. (2019 December 11). *A comprehensive guide to using acids in your skincare routine.* Everyday Health. Health https://www.everydayhealth.com/skin-beauty/a-comprehensive-guide-to-using-acids-in-your-skin-care-routine/

Migala, J. (2019 September 3). *The best skin-care ingredients and products to shield against environmental damage.* Everyday Health. https://www.everydayhealth.com/skin-beauty/how-shield-your-skin-from-environmental-damage/

Montanez, M. (2012 October 9). *10 Ways to celebrate the beauty of women.* Sheknows. https://www.sheknows.com/health-and-wellness/articles/811092/10-ways-to-celebrate-the-beauty-of-women/

Morris, N. (2021 April 8). Why celebrating 'mixed-race beauty' has its problematic side. *The Guardian.* https://www.theguardian.co/commentisfree/2021/apr/08/why-celebrating-mixed-race-beauty-has-its-problematic-side

Mountford, T. (2022 June 29). *2 Treatments to get rid of a turkey neck.* Cosmetic Skin Clinic. https://www.cosmeticskinclinic.com/2018/03/08/2-treatments-to-get-rid-of-a-turkey-neck/

National Association of Ayurvedic Schools and Colleges. (2020 February 12). *Legal status of ayurvedic education in the United States.* https://www.ayurvedanaasc.org/legal-status-of-ayurveda-education/

Nazario, B. (2020 June 25). *Microneedling.* WebMD. https://www.webmd.com/beauty/what_is_microneedling

Nichols, H. (2020 August 10). *Botox: Cosmetic and medical uses.* https://www.medicalnewstoday.com/articles/158647

Nikki. (n.d.). *Hair Removal through the ages: A history of unwanted hair.* A Smooth Life. https://asmoothlife.com/history-hair-removal

North, E. (n.d.). *Effects of alcohol on skin and how to repair the damage.* GoodtoKnow. https://www.goodto.com/wellbeing/effects-of-alcohol-on-skin-396506

Norton, A. (2010 November 10). *White women's skin may show wrinkles sooner.* Reuters Health. https://www.reuters.com/article/us-skin-wrinkles-idUSTRE6A941S20101110

Novolsielski, K., Sipiński, A., Kuczerawy, I. et al. (2012 May 22). Tattoos, piercing, and sexual behaviors in young adults. *The Journal of Sexual Medicine.* https://onlinelibrary.wiley.com/doi/abs/10.1111/j.174 3-6109.2012.02791.x

Nursing Times Contributor. (2017 November 27). Anatomy and physiology of ageing 11: The skin. *Nursing Times.* https://www.nursingtimes.net/roles/older-people-nurses-roles/anatomy-and-physiology-of-ageing-11-the-skin-27-11-2017/

Oakley, A. (2014 June). *What causes acne?* Dermnet NZ. https://dermnetnz.org/topics/what-causes-acne

Oakley, A., Bell, H. (2022 May). *Alopecia areata.* Dermnet NZ. https://dermnetnz.org/topics/alopecia-areata

Oakley, A., Collier, J. (2014 February). *Psychological effects of acne.* DermNet NZ https://dermnetnz.org/topics/psychological-effects-of-acne

Ohyama, M. (2006 December 12). Hair follicle bulge: A fascinating reservoir of epithelial stem cells. *Journal of Dermatological Science.* https://www.jdsjournal.com/article/S0923-1811(06)00359-8/

Okafor, J., (2022 April 23). Environmental impact of cosmetics. *Sustainable Living.* https://www.trvst.world/sustainable-living/environmental-impact-of-cosmetics/

One Planet. (2018 January 30). *The leaping bunny – cruelty-free certification.* https://www.oneplanetnetwork.org/knowledge-centre/resources/leaping-bunny-cruelty-free-certification

Palmer, A. (2020 May 12). *Does oily skin need a moisturizer?* Verywellhealth. https://www.verywellhealth.com/do-i-need-a-moisturizer-if-i-have-oily-skin-15595

Palmer, V. (2022 March 3). *Heavy metal: The benefits of zinc on the skin.* Glowday. https://www.glowday.com/blog/heavy-metal-the-benefits-of-zinc

Palmer, A. (2020 September 20). *Is Retinol the same as Retin-A?* Verywellhealth. https://www.verywellhealth.com/retinol-vs-retin-a-4155865

Palmer, A. (2021 September 13). *Treating acne with Aczone (Dapsone).* Verywellhealth. https://www.verywellhealth.com/aczone-dapsone-15884

Pandey, A., Jatana, G. K., Sonthalia, S. (2021 December 12). Cosmeceuticals. *National Library of Medicine.* https://www.ncbi.nlm.nih.gov/books/NBK544223/

Pandey, M. (2020 July 5). *Why I used skin-whitening products.* BBC News. https://www.bbc.com/news/newsbeat-53275734

Peng, L., Chuo, S. C., Mohd-Nasir, H. et al. (2019 November 13). Role of nanotechnology for design and development of cosmeceutical: Application in Makeup and skin care. *Frontiers in Chemistry.* https://www.frontiersin.org/articles/10.3389/fchem.2019.00739/full

People Pill. (n.d.). *Arthur Hinkel.* https://peoplepill.com/people/arthur-hinkel

Permanence. (n.d.). *Electrolysis History.* https://permanence.com.au/about-electrolysis/electrolysis/history/

Permanence. (n.d.). *Hair removal methods compared.* https://permanence.com.au/about-electrolysis/electrolysis/hair-removal-compared/

Petre, A. (2018 December 19). *What is vegetable glycerin? Uses, benefits and side effects.* Healthline. https://www.healthline.com/nutrition/vegetable-glycerin

Press, L. (2017 March 5). *The ancient secrets of Japanese beauty.* Lemiché Press. https://medium.com/@lemiche/the-ancient-secrets-of-japanese-beauty-be7e90ead114

Prinzivalli, L. & Dancer, R. (2022 April 7). *What is led light therapy and how can it benefit the skin?* Allure. https://www.allure.com/story/what-is-led-light-therapy-skin-benefits

Pruthi, G. K., Babu N. (2012 January - February). Physical and psychological impact of acne in adult females. *Indian Journal of Dermatology.* https://www.ncbi.nlm.nih.gov/pmc/articles/PMC3312651

Purnawamati, S., Indrastuti, N., Danarti, R. et al. (2017 December 15). The role of moisturisers in addressing various kinds of dermatitis: A review. *PubMed Central* https://www.ncbi.nlm.nih.gov/pmc/articles/PMC5849435/

Pyvovarov, S., Spirin, Y. (2022 June 9). *Red lipstick was a symbol of women's struggle for their rights, and during World War 11 it became a weapon for victory over Nazism, as it was hated by Hitler.* Babel. https://babel.ua/en/texts/80004-red-lipstick-was-a-symbol-of-women-s-struggle-for-their-rights-and-during-world-war-ii-it-also-became-a-weapon-for-victory-over-nazism-as-it-was-hated-by-hitler-a-story-in-archival-photos

Rahman, S. (2014 October 3). *How to tackle dark under-eye circles in ethnic skin.* Netdoctor. https://www.netdoctor.co.uk/beauty/a8995/how-to-tackle-dark-under-eye-circles-in-ethnic-skin/

Rawlings, A. V. (2006 March 28). Ethnic skin types: Are there differences in skin structure and function? *International Journal of Cosmetic Science,* Volume 28, Issue 2. https://onlinelibrary.wiley.com/doi/full/10.1111/j.1467-2494.2006.00302.x

Raymond, J. (2021 July 13). *Does drinking water really help your skin?* WebMD. https://www.webmd.com/beauty/features/drink-water-skin

Reece, R. L. (2017 August 8). *Skin tone and racial advantage.* Scalawag. https://scalawagmagazine.org/2017/08/by-the-numbers-skin-tone-and-racial-advantage/

Ricketts, M. (n.d.). *Five skincare ingredients to try.* BirchBox https://www.birchbox.co.uk/features/article/five-skincare-ingredients-to-try

Roberts, W. E. (2009 August 6). Skin type classification systems old and new. *Science Direct.* https://www.sciencedirect.com/sdfe/pdf/download/eid/1-s2.0-S0733863509000540/

Roden, K., Fields, K., Majewski, G. et al. (2016 Descember 14). Skincare Bootcamp: The evolving role of skincare. *PRS Open Global.* https://www.ncbi.nlm.nih.gov/pmc/articles/PMC5172479/

Romm, S. (1987 January 27). Beauty through History. *The Washington Post.* https://www.washingtonpost.com/archive/lifestyle/wellness/1987/01/27/beauty-through-history/

Ross-Hazel, L. (2018 July 10). *What are nails made of?* Healthline. https://www.healthline.com/health/beauty-skin-care/what-are-nails-made-of

Rove, C. (2021 July 2). *Winston Churchill's secret tattoo.* Edenbridge. https://edenbridge.co.uk/blogs/news/winston-churchills-secret-tattoo

Rubin, J. P., (2018). Managing the cosmetic patient. *Plastic Surgery, Volume 2: Aesthetic Surgery.* https://www.sciencedirect.com/topics/psychology/cosmetic-surgery

Saini. (2020 December 24). *Beauty routine smartmirror: Improve your favourite daily task.* Hilo. https://www.hilosmartmirror.com/beauty-routine-smart-mirror/

Sakai, S., Yasuda, R., Sayo, T. et al. (2000 June). Hyaluronic acid exists in the normal stratum corneum. *PubMed.gov.* https://pubmed.ncbi.nlm.nih.gov/10844564

Salvioni, L., Morelli, L., Ochoa, E. et al. (2021 July). The emerging role of nanotechnology in skincare. *ScienceDirect.*

*https://www.sciencedirect.com/science/article/pii/S000186862
1000786*

Sampson, S. (2019 November 1). *Is it normal to shed this much?*
Greatist. https://greatist.com/

Santos-Longhurst, A. (2021 August 20). *Understanding and
managing chronic inflammation.* Healthline.
https://www.healthline.com/health/chronic-
inflammation

Saved Tattoo. (2022 April 19). *How deep should a tattoo needle go?*
https://www.savedtattoo.com/how-deep-should-a-
tattoo-needle-go/

Scheve, T. (2021 April 8). *How many muscles does it take to smile?*
HowStuffWorks.
https://science.howstuffworks.com/life/inside-the-
mind/emotions/muscles-smile.htm

Scott, E. (2021 October 7). *The link between stress and adult acne.*
VeryWellMind. https://www.verywellmind.com/does-
stress-cause-acne-3144829

Scripps. (2020 November 23). *How to fix turkey neck with plastic
surgery.* https://www.scripps.org/news_items/7103-
how-to-fix-turkey-neck-with-plastic-surgery

Sherrell, Z. (2021 June 29). *What can damage the subcutaneous layer?*
MedicalNewsToday.
https://www.medicalnewstoday.com/articles/subcutan
eous-layer

Silverthorne, S. (2010 April 19). *The History of Beauty.* Harvard
Business School. https://hbswk.hbs.edu/item/the-
history-of-beauty

Simms, S. (2015 January 14). *Lead, mercury and death: Beauty's historically high cost.* Allthatsinteresting. https://allthatsinteresting.com/makeup-history

Sinha, S. (2022 January 4). *Tetracycline.* Drugs.com. https://www.drugs.com/tetracycline.html

Sivak, H. (2015 June 17). *Solvents.* https://hannahsivak.com/blog/solvents/

Smith, A. (2021 September 3). *How do people from different racial groups age?* MedicalNewsToday. https://www.medicalnewstoday.com/articles/how-different-races-age

Smith, J. (2020 May 14). *How do processed foods affect your health?* MedicalNewsToday https://www.medicalnewstoday.com/articles/318630

Smith, M. (2020 August 24). *Pustules.* WebMD. https://www.webmd.com/skin-problems-and-treatments/guide/pustules-fact

Snowperk (n.d.). *Understanding the 8 classifications of your resistant skin types.* https://snowperk.com/blog/understanding-the-8-classifications-of-your-resistant-skin-type/

Sood, S. (2012 November 30). *The origins of bathhouse culture around the world.* BBC Travel. https://www.bbc.com/travel/article/20121129-the-origins-of-bathhouse-culture-around-the-world

Spritzer, P.M., Barone, C. R., De Oliveira, F. B. ((2016 December). Hirsutism in polycystic ovary syndrome: Pathophysiology and management. *PubMed.* https://pubmed.ncbi.nlm.nih.gov/27510481/

Stocum, D. L., (2013). Hair Follicle. *Handbook of Stem Cells,* (Second Edition) https://www.sciencedirect.com/topics/engineering/hair-follicle

Strong, R. (2022 March 31). *Hoping to even out your skin tone? Tranexamic acid could help.* Healthline. https://www.healthline.com/health/beauty-skin-care/tranexamic-acid-for-skin

Stuart, A. (2021 October 13). *What's your skin type?* WebMD. https://webmd.com/beauty/whats-your-skin-type

Style Story. (2021 December 13). *How to layer acids in your skincare routine.* https://stylestory.com.au/blogs/style-story/how-to-layer-acids-in-your-skincare-routine

Summers, G. (2022 February 16). *Everything you ever wanted to know about petroleum jelly for the skin.* Byrdie. https://www.byrdie.com/is-petroleum-jelly-safe-2442885

Sweet, J. (2021 December 28). *11 Skincare myths you should stop believing, according to dermatologists.* Forbes. https://www.forbes.com/sites/jonisweet/2021/12/28/11-skincare-myths-you-should-stop-believing-according-to-dermatologists/?sh=4c9664de3611

Syed, F. (2019) December 3). *How your face will age.* Slice Canada. https://www.slice.ca/how-your-face-will-age-based-on-race-according-to science/

Takeao, M., Lee, W. & Ito, M. (2015). *Wound healing and skin regeneration.* The Ronald O. Perelman Department of Dermatology, New York University, School of Medicine New York. Cold Spring Harbour Laboratory Press. https://www.woundsworld.com/wp-content/uploads/2021/02/Wound-Healing-and-Skin-Regeneration.pdf

Tan, J. K. L., Bhate, K. (2015 July). A global perspective on the epidemiology of acne. *The British Journal of Dermatology.* PubMed https://pubmed.ncbi.nlm.nih.gov/25597339

Tariemi, O. (2022 January 27). *Otjize: The red beauty miracle of the Himba people.* Life. https://guardian.ng/life/otjize-the-red-beauty-miracle-of-the-himba-people/

Taylor Hays, J. (2020 November 19). *Is it true that smoking causes wrinkles?* Mayo Clinic. https://www.mayoclinic.org/healthy-lifestyle/quit-smoking/expert-answers/smoking/faq-20058153

Team Linchpin. (2022 January 13). *Trends shaping the future of beauty and cosmetics in 2022.* https://linchpinseo.com/trends-beauty-and-cosmetics/

Tectales. (2018 October 17). *3D Printng cells to produce human tissue.* https://tectales.com/3d-printing/3d-printing-cells-to-produce-human-tissue.html

Thayers (n.d.). *The importance of dermatologist-tested skincare products.* https://www.thayers.com/the-importance-of-dermatologist-tested-skincare.html

The Guardian. (2021 March 17). Investing in Africa: *Why beauty companies are swarming in.* https://guardian.ng/features/investing-in-africa-why-beauty-companies-are-swarming-in/

Thompson, K. (2021 January 20). *'Beauty is your duty' 80 years on - Churchill's campaign that would spark outrage today.* The Daily Mirror. https://www.mirror.co.uk/news/uk-news/beauty-your-duty-80-years-23355838

Thomas, M. (2021 July 222). *What to know about blue light screen protectors.* MedicalNewsToday. https://www.medicalnewstoday.com/articles/best-blue-light-screen-protectors

Timmens, J.& Editorial Team Healthline. (2022 February 4). *Age Spots.* Healthline. https://www.healthline.com/health/age-spotshttps://www.uni-europa.org/sectors/hair-beauty/

Toogood, S. (2022 July 21).Email.

Trevino, J. (2018 October 12). *Glowing skin might start in your genes.* Popular Science. https://www.popsci.com/genetics-skin-health/

Turner, N. (2014 September 11). *Fighting aging and look younger by balancing your hormones.* Chatelaine. https://www.chatelaine.com/health/diet/fight-aging-and-look-younger-by-balancing-your-hormones/

UK Reach. (2021 September 3). *UK Reach − restriction proposals 002 − Call for evidence: substances in tattoo inks and permanent make-up* (PMU). https://consultations.hse.gov.uk/crd-reach/restriction-proposals-002/

Uni Europa Hair & Beauty. (n.d.). *Sectors: Hair and beauty.* Uni Global Union Europa. https://www.uni-europa.org/sectors/hair-beauty/

Unilever. (n.d.). *Vaseline healthy skin, every day.* https://www.unileverusa.com/brands/beauty-wellbeing/vaseline/

Ursin, F., Borelli, C. &Steger, F. (2019 September 21). Dermatology in Ancient Rome: Medical ingredients in Ovid's 'Remedies for female faces.'. *Journal of Cosmetic Dermatology.*

https://onlinelibrary.wiley.com/doi/full/10.1111/jocd.
13151

USDA. (2022). *Organic Agriculture USA.*
https://www.gov.uk/guidance/organic-food-uk-
approved-control-bodies

USSEC. (2016 July 25). *Research suggests soy isoflavones may help
promote skin health.* US Soybean Export Council.
https://ussec.org/research-suggests-soy-isoflavones-
may-help-promote-skin-health/

Vacarro, C. M. (2010). *The New Wellness: When beauty means
health.*
https://ideas.repec.org/a/mul/j1t56u/doi10.2382-
32700y2010i1p91-102.html

Vandergriendt, C. (2019 September 12). *What's the difference
between UVA and UVB rays?* Healthline.
https://www.healthline.com/health/skin/uva-vs-
uvb#bottom-line

Villines, Z., Sharon, A. (2021 November 30). *Causes of unwanted
hair growth (hirsutism).* MedicalNewsToday.
https://www.medicalnewstoday.com/articles/323540

VR Foundation (n.d.). *About Vitiligo.*
https://vrfoundation.org/about_vitiligo

Walters, M. (2022 February 11). *Boost your skin's regeneration
process for a glowing, vibrant complexion.* Healthline.
https://www.healthline.com/health/skin-regeneration

Wan, D. C., Wong, V. W., Longaker, M. T. et al. (2014 June 7).
Moisturizing different racial skin types. *The Journal of
Clinical and Aesthetic Dermatology.*
https://www.ncbi.nlm.nih.gov/pmc/articles/PMC4086
530/

WebMD. (2020). *Collagen peptides - uses, side effects, and more.* WebMD. https://www/webmd.com/vitamins/ai/ingredientmon o-1606/collagen-peptides

WebMD. (2010 March 1). *The Science of hair.* WebMD. https://www.webmd.com/skin-problems-and-treatments/hair-loss/science-hair

WebMD Editorial Contributors. (2021 June 28). *What is a humectant?* WebMD. https://www.webmd.com/skin-problems-and-treatments/what-is-a-humectant

Whitbread, L. (2017 December 19). *Beauty slang words meaning.* Refinery 29. https://www.refinery29.com/en-us/2017/12/186061/beauty-slang-term-words-meaning

Whitten, C. (20121 November 22). *What to know about ayurvedic skincare.* WebMD. https://www.webmd.com/beauty/what-to-know-about-ayurvedic-skin-care

Wikipedia. (n.d.). *Havelock Ellis.* https://en.wikipedia.org/wiki/Havelock_Ellis

Wizemann, S. (2020 December 28). *What you need to know about occlusives in skincare.* Good Housekeeping Institute. https://www.goodhousekeeping.com/beauty-products/a34406550/what-is-occlusive-skincare-ingredients/

Wolters Kluwer Health. (2019 January 30). *What causes aging of the upper lip? Loss of volume, not just sagging.* ScienceDaily. https://www.sciencedaily.com/releases/2019/01/1901 30133040.htm

Woodside, P. (2017 April 15). *Difference between glycolic acid & glycerin.* Sciencing. https://sciencing.com/differences-between-glycolic-acid-glycerin-8062972.html

World Health Organization Fact sheet. (2022 May 9). *Alcohol.* https://www.who.int/news-room/fact-sheets/detail/alcohol

Yahoo. (2021 December 24). *7 Alcoholic drinks ranked from bad to worst for your skin.* https://uk.style.yahoo.com/7-alcoholic-drinks-ranked-bad-094000613.html?

Yang, A. (2020 September 15). Ancient DNA is revealing the genetic landscape of people who first settled East Asia. *The Conversation.* https://theconversation.com/ancient-dna-is-revealing-the-genetic-landscape-of-people-who-first-settled-east-asia-139458

Yang, E. (2021 September 22). *The 9 types of protein derms and RDs recommended eating for healthy, glowing skin.* Well + Good. https://www.wellandgood.com/protein-for-healthy-skin/

Yang, J., Yang, H., Xu, A. et al. (2020 September 17). A review of advancement on influencing factors of acne: An emphasis on environmental characteristics. *Frontiers in Public Health.* https://www.ncbi.nlm.nih.gov/pmc/articles/PMC7527424/

Yetman, D. (2020 July 17). *What is radiofrequency skin tightening?* Healthline. https://www.healthline.com/health/beauty-skin-care/radio-frequency-skin-tightening

Yoo-jeong, L., Ji-woo, C. & Sae-young, S. (2020 December). A Study on the direction of evaluation indicators for personalised beauty self-care. *Journal of Fashion Business,*

Volume   24   Edition   6.
http://www.koreascience.or.kr/article/JAKO20200715
9775478.j

Zarrelli, N. (2016 November 21). This advice column from Victorian England shows how women poisoned themselves in the name of beauty. *Business Insider.* https://www.businessinsider.com/this-advice-column-from-victorian-england-shows-how-women-poisoned-themselves-in-the-name-of-beauty-2016-10

Zhao, L., Hu, M., Xiao, Q. et al. (2021 July 16). Efficacy and safety of platelet-rich plasma in melasma: A systematic review and meta-analysis. *Dermatology and Therapy. https://link.springer.com/article/10.1007/s13555-021-00575-z*

Zouboullis, C. C., Blume-Peytavi, U., Kosmadaki, M. et al. (2022 February 25). Skin, hair and beyond: The impact of menopause. *Climeteric.* https://www.tandfonline.com/doi/full/10.1080/13697137.2022.2050206?src=recsys

Images

All images sourced from istockphoto.com.

About the Authors

Katie Lewis obtained her qualification of City & Guilds NVQ Level 2 & 3 in Electrolysis and Beauty Therapy at Ware Regional College in 1995. She has since acquired many hours of experience in all areas of beauty therapy.

Katie runs her own business in Hertfordshire, specialising in electrolysis. She is a member of the British Association of Electrolysis.

Katie found her true passion in life helping people overcome serious confidence issues with unwanted hair. She helps people who suffer from Polycystic Ovary Syndrome (PCOS), which unfortunately creates Hirsutism (male-pattern hair growth on a woman's face, chest, and back). She also specialises in helping transgender people with their transition, as hair removal is vital in this process. Katie has hundreds of happy customers and reviews. (https://katielewis.uk)

Jarrett Zapletal is passionate about a healthy lifestyle and food. He is a chef experimenting with international cuisines and a pescatarian. He uses nearly exclusively homegrown organic vegetables and herbs. He is a herbalist, author, and spiritualist and confesses he is a gym addict.

Jarrett has a lifelong interest in skincare, and he secretly started using his mother's creams at the age of 13. To this day he regularly receives compliments on how much younger he looks than his actual age.

Intensely interested in history and philosophy, he delved deep into the roots of the beauty trade and discovered that beauty is more than skin deep. He believes that beauty has a spiritual dimension which enriches lives and contributes to emotional well-being.

Jarrett grew up in the former Czechoslovakia, where his family still makes award-winning wines.

Today this region is a UNESCO biosphere reserve, but to his grandparents it was the 'land burned by sun', as their ancestors called it since the beginning of human settlements. They lived according to the seasons and Jarrett remembered irises, sandwort, Mediterranean sages, and alpine oatgrass blooming on the karst forest steppe, a unique transitional eco-system between Europe and Asia.

Jarrett remembers the rituals in his grandparents' homes. They are firmly cemented into his memory: His grandfather was up at 04:30 in the morning, working the lands till sunset with unwavering energy. His grandmother's features were soft in the filtered light of the net curtains, while chopping onions and herbs for the Knödels (dumplings). The rituals of their days – early to bed, spring water, fresh food without any chemicals, hard work on their small farm – brought them comfort and, in spite of political turmoil, a sense of belonging to their descendants.

He often wonders whether these memories shaped his art as he travelled across Europe and Morocco to the British Isles. He now lives in the British countryside, still trying to catch the essence of beauty in his art – even in the imperfect. He records the fleeting moments where people, unaware of the comfort their rituals bring them, go about their daily lives.

In this book, Jarrett and Katie collaborated to bring their knowledge and experience of many years together for a unique insight into the beauty industry.